Synthesis Lectures on Visualization

Series Editors

This series publishes on topics pertaining to scientific visualization, information visualization, and visual analytics. Potential topics include, but are not limited to scientific, information, and medical visualization; visual analytics, applications of visualization and analysis; mathematical foundations of visualization and analytics; interaction, cognition, and perception related to visualization and analytics; data integration, analysis, and visualization; new applications of visualization and analysis; knowledge discovery management and representation; systems, and evaluation; distributed and collaborative visualization and analysis.

Katarína Furmanová · Barbora Kozlíková ·
Thomas Höllt · M. Eduard Gröller ·
Bernhard Preim · Renata Georgia Raidou

BioMedical Visualization

Past Work, Current Trends, and Open Challenges

Springer

Katarína Furmanová
Faculty of Informatics
Masaryk University
Brno, Czech Republic

Barbora Kozlíková
Faculty of Informatics
Masaryk University
Brno, Czech Republic

Thomas Höllt
Faculty of Electrical Engineering
Mathematics and Computer Science
Delft University of Technology
Delft, The Netherlands

M. Eduard Gröller
Institute of Visual Computing
and Human-Centered Technology
TU Wien
Wien, Austria

Bernhard Preim
Faculty of Computer Science
Otto von Guericke University Magdeburg
Magdeburg, Germany

Renata Georgia Raidou
Institute of Visual Computing
and Human-Centered Technology
TU Wien
Wien, Austria

ISSN 2159-516X ISSN 2159-5178 (electronic)
Synthesis Lectures on Visualization
ISBN 978-3-031-66791-6 ISBN 978-3-031-66789-3 (eBook)
https://doi.org/10.1007/978-3-031-66789-3

This Springer imprint is published by the registered company Springer Nature Switzerland AG
The registered company address is: Gewerbestrasse 11, 6330 Cham, Switzerland

Preface

Medicine and biology are important research fields with a significant impact on humans and their health. In the last few decades, many visualization strategies have been proposed for solving problems within these disciplines. From the early molecular models and medical volume representations to modern-day visual analytics for genomics or extended reality applications for surgery training and guidance, the area of biomedical visualization has progressed and expanded considerably.

The goal of this book is to provide an overview of biomedical visualization by highlighting the overall trends of research through the years and the evolution of topics over time. To uncover these trends, we have manually curated a total of 3856 research publications related to biomedical visualization, which we categorized according to their application field. A searchable repository of these publications accompanies this book at https://biomedvis-book.fi.muni.cz/.

The topics we cover in this book include visualization research in omics, interaction networks and pathways, biological structures, tumor diagnosis and treatment, vasculature, brain, surgery, educational contexts, therapy and rehabilitation, electronic health records, and public health. A separate chapter is dedicated to general visualization techniques commonly used for biomedical data, such as surface and volume rendering, as well as abstract and illustrative approaches. For each of these areas, the past and contemporary research trends are discussed, highlighting the most influential works. Furthermore, the book explains how research is affected by developments in technology, data availability, and domain practice.

Moreover, we discuss visualization challenges that can be considered solved, as well as research directions anticipated to thrive in the upcoming years. We further include the outcomes of interviews conducted with 16 researchers in the field of biomedical visualization to solicit their opinions regarding the evolution and trends in the domain as well as the future of this research field.

We discuss the individual topics in a concise manner to help readers orient themselves in the already mature and diverse field of biomedical visualization without overwhelming them with technical details. We also provide useful pointers for future reading. As such, we hope that the book can help young researchers to become familiar with past challenges and identify future ones. For more senior researchers, we believe our book can serve as an insightful overview of the research field and the direction it is heading.

We invite you to join us on our journey through the research history of BioMedical Visualization and hope you will enjoy reading this book.

Brno, Czech Republic — Katarína Furmanová
Brno, Czech Republic — Barbora Kozlíková
Delft, The Netherlands — Thomas Höllt
Wien, Austria — M. Eduard Gröller
Magdeburg, Germany — Bernhard Preim
Wien, Austria — Renata Georgia Raidou
May 2024

Acknowledgements

When we set out to map the field of BioMedical Visualization, we had little idea of the journey that awaited us. Here we would like to express our gratitude to the people, who made this work possible. Firstly, a big "thank you" to our families and friends for their constant support and understanding. A special acknowledgment goes to Martin Steller (TU Wien) for implementing the searchable repository that accompanies this work available at https://biomedvis-book.fi.muni.cz/. We also thank the 16 researchers (wishing to remain anonymous) who enriched this book with their insights and experiences in written interviews which we present in one of the book chapters. Our work was also shaped by feedback from reviewers and colleagues. We thank them for providing us with helpful advice which enabled us to improve this book. Finally, we would also like to thank our institutions for supporting us in our work: Masaryk University, Delft University of Technology, Otto von Guericke University of Magdeburg, TU Wien, and VRVis, which is funded by BMK, BMDW, Styria, SFG, Tyrol and Vienna Business Agency in the scope of COMET—Competence Centers for Excellent Technologies (879730) which is managed by FFG.

Contents

1 Introduction

Biological and medical visualization has been a growing research area for several decades. Through the years, many visualization strategies have been designed and the focus of the field has been changing and adapting to new challenges that arose over time. This book is intended to provide a comprehensive and structured overview of *BioVis*, e.g., molecular visualization and metabolic pathway visualization, and *MedVis*, e.g., 3D visualizations for diagnosis, treatment, and education. While some topics clearly belong to either BioVis or MedVis, there are also overlaps among the two domains. For example, the analysis of microscopic images at a cellular level integrates BioVis techniques, such as image analysis of sub-cellular components, with MedVis aspects, such as developing systems for supporting clinical workflows. In the context of this book, we refer to these techniques—*BioVis*, *MedVis*, or "in-between"—as *BioMedical Visualization*.

BioMedical Visualization has been an enabler for medical diagnosis and treatment and an influential component of today's life science research. Many BioMedical domains can now be studied at various scales and dimensions, employing different acquisition modalities and simulations, and supporting various purposes—from genomic to public health data, and from biomolecules to large-scale volumes.

This book is motivated by the maturity of BioVis and MedVis after several decades of intense research worldwide. Due to the growth of the field, it has meanwhile become very challenging for Ph.D. students and industrial researchers to oversee the area. After the publication of focused state-of-the-art reviews on special BioVis and MedVis topics, such as visual computing for radiation treatment planning [551], visual analytics for public health [485], and visualization of biomolecular structures [320], we aim to provide a broader picture.

We observe that throughout the history of BioMedical Visualization, there have been three interesting tendencies. Firstly, *advances of the visualization field* progress along with

K. Furmanová et al., *BioMedical Visualization*, Synthesis Lectures on Visualization,
https://doi.org/10.1007/978-3-031-66789-3_1

imaging modalities, such as the visualization of the multiscale, multimodal, cohort, or computational biology data, as well as the emergence of Visual Analytics with the increasing incorporation of artificial intelligence and "human-in-the-loop" concepts. Secondly, we witness the *re-emergence of topics* once every few years, such as the use of augmented and virtual reality for educational purposes. Thirdly, research makes its way *from general towards more specialized solutions*. While in the past, general solutions were developed (e.g., vessel visualization or virtual endoscopy), nowadays research tends towards special problems or diseases (e.g., aneurysms).

With this book, we set out to answer the following questions: *What are the overall trends through the years? How are the topics evolving with the course of time? Where is the field heading in the upcoming decade?* Our book aims to make the following **contributions**:

- an extensive historical search of the papers related to BioMedical Visualization;
- a taxonomy of BioMedical Visualization, i.e., of the topics and the people/groups working on these, along the course of time;
- a characterization of more than 3,800 papers, and
- an online, interactive repository accompanying the book, where our collection of papers and taxonomy is made available to the community for further use at https://biomedvis-book.fi.muni.cz/.

1.1 Literature Search and Scope

The book has an unusually broad scope, leading us to consider more than 3,800 publications. This broad scope poses several challenges with regard to the extent of the search and the resulting taxonomy. We conducted an extensive search of literature databases, using consistently the following search term to discover previous work in visualization, visual analytics, and augmented and virtual reality on recurrent topics or applications in BioVis and MedVis:

```
("molecular" OR "biological" OR "medical" OR
"anatomical" OR "biomolecular" OR "biochemical" OR
"chemical" OR "biomedical" OR "bioinformatics" OR
"biomechanics" OR "cell" OR "cellular" OR "microbiology"
OR "genetics" OR "histology" OR "pathology" OR
"histopathology" OR "neuroscience" OR "pharmacology" OR
"physiology" OR "surgical") AND ("visualization" OR
"visualisation" OR "visual analytics" OR "visual
computing" OR "visual analysis" OR "virtual reality" OR
"augmented reality" OR "mixed reality" OR "graphics" OR
"human computer interaction")
```

For the literature search, we considered the sources in Table 1.1. When possible, e.g., in PubMed or IEEE Xplore, logical search operators were used to directly apply the aforementioned search term. Otherwise, e.g., in the Eurographics Digital Library, where the search is limited, the considered journals or proceedings were reviewed manually on a one-to-one basis. The searches were not filtered with regard to publication time and all years were considered—spanning even back to 1969 until April 2024. In IEEE Xplore, an initial search

Table 1.1 Sources and respective numbers of identified papers

Source	Papers
IEEE Transactions on Visualization and Computer Graphics (TVCG)	386
EG DigLib (excl. EG VCBM and CGF)	276
EG Visual Computing in Biology and Medicine (VCBM)	261
Computer Graphics Forum (CGF)	240
Computers and Graphics (C&G)	193
IEEE VIS and SciVis	167
IEEE Computer Graphics and Applications (CGA)	134
IEEE Information Visualization (IV)	122
Bioinformatics	101
IEEE Virtual Reality (VR)	98
BMC Bioinformatics	92
International Journal of Computer Assisted Radiology and Surgery (JCars)	74
The Visual Computer	70
IEEE ISMAR	58
IEEE PacificVis	55
Nature (Methods, Biotechnology, Communications, ...)	53
IEEE Access	52
IEEE Visual Analytics in Healthcare (VAHC)	46
ACM SIGGRAPH, SIGGRAPH Asia	45
IEEE Symposium on BioVis	45
IEEE Trans. on Medical Imaging (TMI)	44
IEEE Trans. on Biomedical Engineering (TBE)	42
Book Sections (Springer)	40
Graphics Interfaces (GI)	26
IEEE Visual Analytics Science & Technology (VAST)	26
Nucleic Acids Research	25
ACM Virtual Reality Software & Technology (VRST)	22
Other various	1063
Total	**3856**

yielded more than 70,000 results. Therefore, we decided not to search the entire database, but to restrict the search to the most significant sources, which are indicated in Table 1.1. For the easy storage and further management of the findings, we used reference management software to manage bibliographic data and related materials. This allowed us to import all relevant works easily, check for duplicates, and further identify out-of-scope works.

Papers, where the term visualization was used to denote pure imaging or processing methods, data mining or data management tools, databases, simple plots of findings, or packages with standard viewers (e.g., in R), were discarded. Only works with a core visualization, visual analytics, or virtual/augmented reality focus were considered. Results were also considered out of scope if they only matched the search term due to titles in the reference list or author biographies, and if they were not within our specific BioVis and MedVis scope. We also restricted our search to papers written in English. The initial search yielded more than 4,000 candidates, which were reduced to 3,856 during a second thorough pass conducted iteratively by multiple co-authors. The numbers in Table 1.1 are those resulting from this second pass. As a companion to this book, which contains only 690 selected key publications, a searchable website with all publications we analyzed is provided at https://biomedvis-book.fi.muni.cz/.

Figure 1.1 shows the number of the considered BioMedVis papers published across time overall (a) and for six prominent venues (b). Since the data for the year 2024 were incomplete at the time of publication, we only included data up to the year 2023 in the timeline graphs in the book. It can be noted, that there is a sudden spike from 172 papers in 2018, to 416 in 2019, and to 337 in 2020, which can be justified by the appearance of a multitude of papers that deal with multimodal, multi-parametric, multi-subject, multiscale data, as well as a multitude of contributions in the fields of rehabilitation (also with VR/AR), omics, and molecular visualization.

1.2 Taxonomy: Overview and Dimensions

Our taxonomy is built upon five dimensions, as illustrated in Fig. 1.2. Given the vast number of papers covered in this book, it is unfeasible to follow a method-based taxonomy. This would yield an unmanageable number of distinct categories, which would not be comparable to each other. We, therefore, decided to focus on general characteristics that are present in all kinds of visualization designs: the **data**, the **stakeholders**, the **tasks**, the **scale**, and the **application field**. For the manual categorization of the literature based on the aforementioned five dimensions, the authors read all abstracts (if this was not sufficient, also the papers) and decided on a one-to-one basis how to categorize them. During the categorization, we also considered the integration of information regarding the evolution and how topics have formed, disappeared, and/or re-emerged since 1969, when the oldest included paper was published. Figure 1.3 depicts the distribution of papers for the five dimensions of the manual categorization.

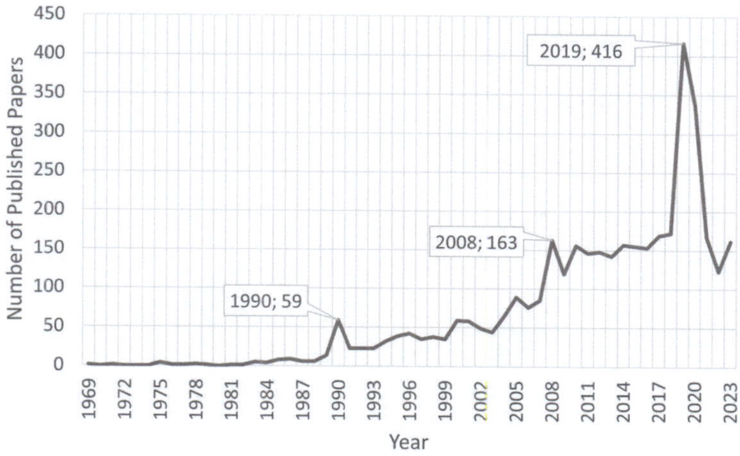

(a)

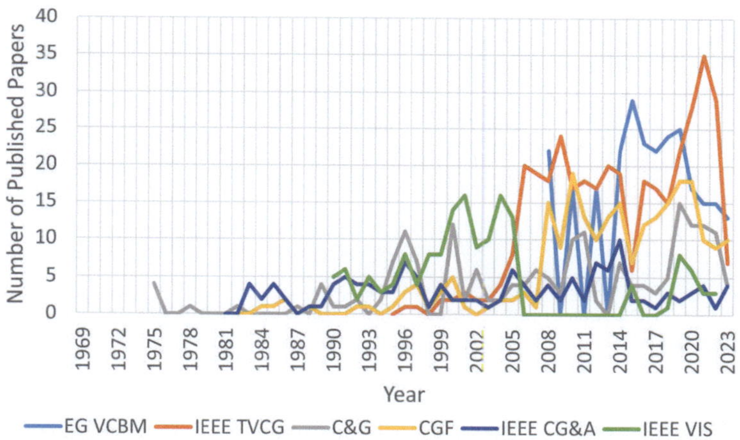

(b)

Fig. 1.1 Number of BioMedVis papers published across time (a) overall; and (b) for six prominent venues: IEEE TVCG, IEEE CGA, CGF, C&G, EG VCBM, IEEE VIS (note that since 2006 most IEEE VIS papers are published in TVCG)

1.3 Outline

The book is structured as follows: Chap. 2 includes prominent techniques used in the field of BioMedical Visualization, while in Chap. 3, we discuss topics within BioMedical Visualization from an application-driven perspective. Subsequent to this we also provide a chapter with position statements, i.e., "undocumented" information about the evolution of

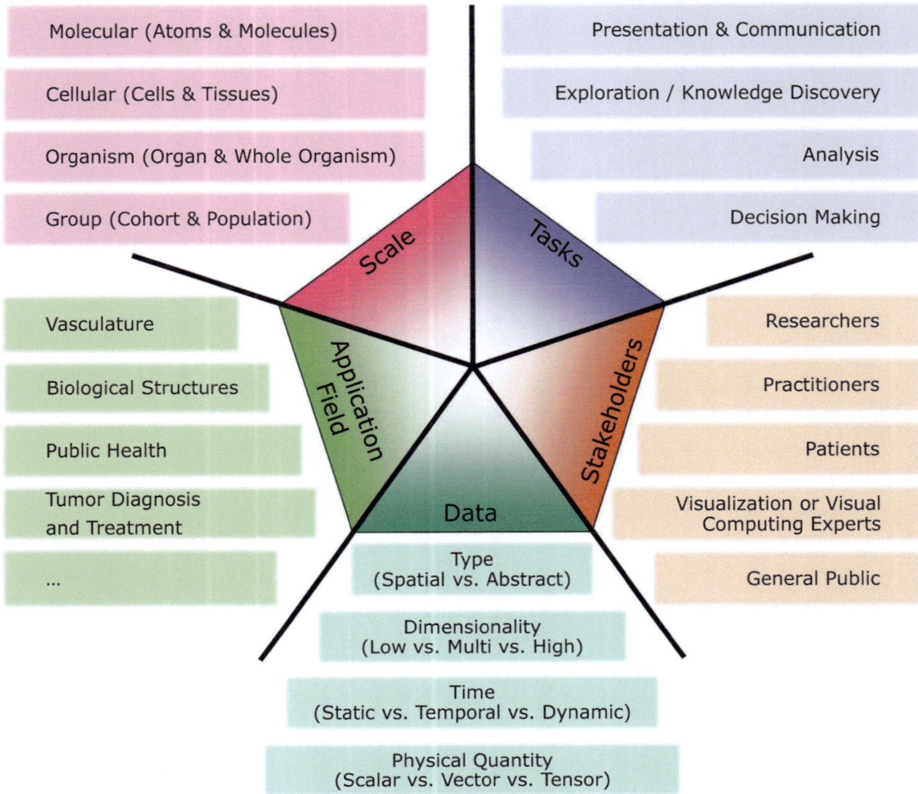

Fig. 1.2 The five dimensions of our taxonomy: the **data**, the **stakeholders**, the **tasks**, the **scale**, and the **application field**

the community, which have been obtained from interviews with 16 BioMedical Visualization researchers (Chap. 4). This is followed by a discussion (Chap. 5), where we examine the present and future challenges. In this chapter, we also employ a natural language processing (NLP) methodology to automatically assess the proposed characterization of previous work and the underlying trends in addition to the manual classification of papers according to our taxonomy. Chapter 6 concludes this book with insights for the future.

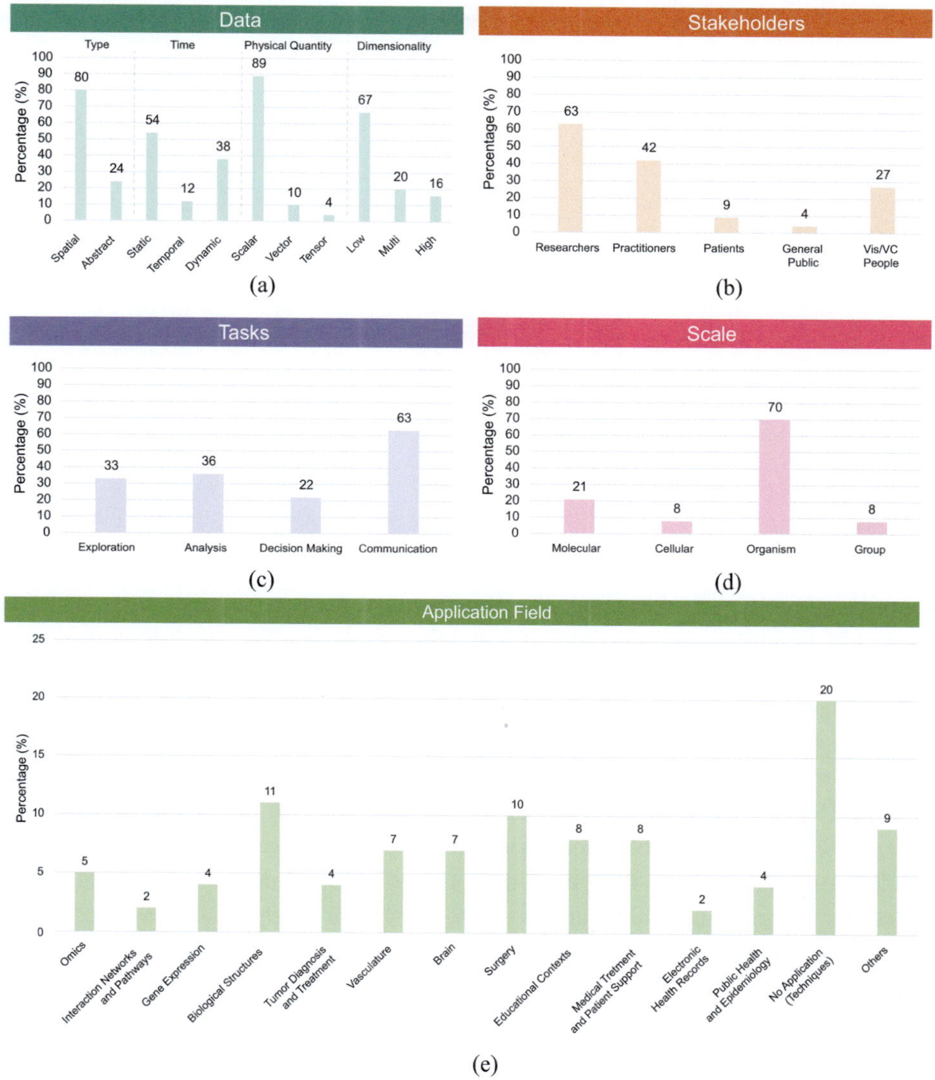

Fig. 1.3 Distribution of papers throughout the five dimensions of the manual categorization: (a) data, (b) stakeholders, (c) tasks, (d) scale of application, and (e) application field. In each graph, the percentages do not sum up to 100%, as some papers might have been assigned to several categories

Techniques

2

A large corpus of the literature we analyzed involved purely technical contributions without a specific application field in mind. Therefore, we first focus on an overview of the most commonly used techniques in BioMedVis and their evolution. We also include references to important surveys that cover each of the discussed topics in greater detail.

According to Fig. 2.1, the earliest general techniques started appearing in the 1980s with significant growth in number in the 1990s. These earliest techniques form the basic building blocks of the medical visualization pipeline and are covered in the surveys on medical imaging [155, 537] and volume visualization and rendering [78]. In the 2000s, we can still see a growing number of publications, which reached the highest numbers at the turn of the decade. Many of the papers from this time focus on GPU-accelerated techniques [53]. In subsequent years we see a slight decline in the number of purely technique-based papers, which is in contrast with trends from individual application fields where we can usually observe an uptake in the 2010s. This is in line with our observation that in the past decade, BioMedVis research has been turning from general multi-purpose techniques to narrowly focused application-oriented solutions.

Rendering algorithms utilized for 3D medical image data were compared by Tiede et al. [620] and by Meißner et al. [401]. The optimization aspect, which mostly concerns GPU utilization in volume rendering for large-scale datasets, has been summarized by Beyer et al. [53]. They categorize existing approaches according to the desired output: ray-guided, visualization-driven, or display-aware techniques. Functional aspects, such as the adjustment of the rendering and its visibility parameters using *transfer functions*, have been reviewed by Arens and Domik [22]. Later, Ljung et al. [382] revised the state of research in transfer functions.

Annotating and labeling of 3D models was summarized in several surveys, as well. Ropinski et al. [526] surveyed glyph-based visualization techniques for exploring spatial

K. Furmanová et al., *BioMedical Visualization*, Synthesis Lectures on Visualization,
https://doi.org/10.1007/978-3-031-66789-3_2

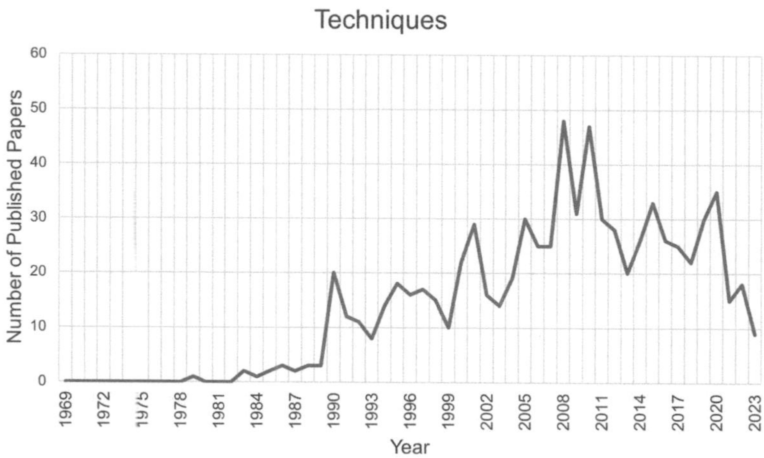

Fig. 2.1 Number of *Technique* papers (i.e., papers without specific application domain) published over time

multivariate medical data, e.g., anatomical data along with functional information or simulation results. Glyphs may be used, for example, to reveal the properties of diffusion tensor data [301] or to reveal simulation information on top of the heart surface. Their classification considers perceptual issues and, thus, they discuss glyphs that support pre-attentive and attentive processing. Glyph design has two essential aspects: the mapping process, where data are mapped to parameters of the glyph shape and appearance, and *glyph placement*, i.e., the decision where to actually render glyphs. Since glyph-based visualizations are not intuitive, a carefully designed glyph legend is essential to convey the mapping.

Conversely, Oeltze-Jafra and Preim [452] reviewed approaches to label medical datasets and classified them according to individual types of labeling techniques (Fig. 2.2). The most essential distinction is between *internal labels* that are displayed on top of anatomical structures, and *external labels* that are placed beyond the anatomical structures and are connected to them via lines. Oeltze-Jafra and Preim also compiled guidelines for choosing an appropriate technique for a given data representation.

Uncertainty in data acquisition and processing is a substantial problem in many research fields. In biology and medicine, it can have significant consequences. Special attention to handling uncertainty has been given in these fields in the last decade. Ristovski et al. [518] investigated the sources of uncertainty in medical visualization and the existing approaches. Furthermore, they identified several open visualization challenges. Later, Linsen et al. [380] discussed sources of uncertainty at different stages of the medical visualization pipeline and provided the readers with means to mathematically describe uncertainty in a medical context. A review focusing on uncertainty-aware visualization in medical imaging has been done by Gillmann et al. [191].

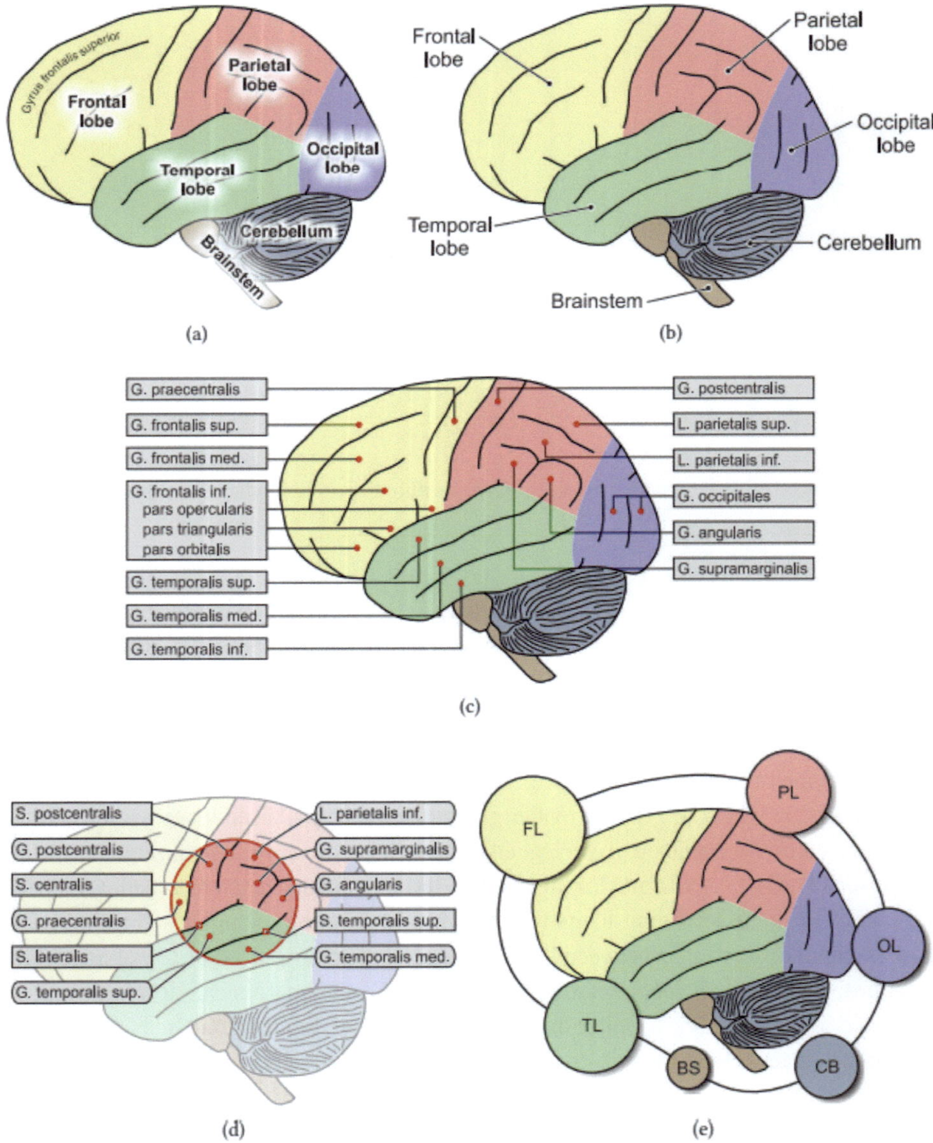

Fig. 2.2 Overview of labeling techniques in medical visualizations: (a) internal, (b) external, (c) boundary, (d) excentric, (e) necklace label placement [452]. *© 2014 The Author(s), Eurographics Proceedings © 2014 The Eurographics Association. Reproduced by kind permission of the Eurographics Association*

Visual perception and aesthetic appearance of representations in biology and medicine are also investigated. An example is volumetric illumination, as surveyed by Jönsson et al. [277]. This work discusses different aspects of illumination techniques: technical realization, performance, and perceptual capabilities. Perceptually motivated 3D visualizations of medical image data have been summarized by Preim et al. [483]. Surface models extracted from medical image data provide opportunities for visual, aesthetic, and perceptual enhancements. For example, Lawonn et al. [354, 356] described various approaches to apply feature lines on medical surface models and surface-based illustrative rendering for visualization. Alternative methods for the visual exploration of complex 3D objects, such as surface flattening approaches, are popular in many applications (e.g., vascular, orthopedic, or endoscopic ones) [321]. Recently, medical animations have also emerged as an important research direction [486]. Animations may be used to convey the dynamics of medical image data, such as perfusion data or measured blood flow (over time). Animations may also be used to convey static 3D data such that a virtual camera sequentially emphasizes different portions of a complex dataset, e.g., for surgery planning.

In *molecular visualization*, essential summaries of the existing approaches were published by Kozlíková et al. [320] and Krone et al. [325]. Alharbi et al. [16] surveyed molecular visualization of computational biology data. The latter work aims to bridge the gap between the visualization and computational domains by presenting links and differences between studies published in both communities.

Finally, *mixed-reality* solutions in the biomedical domain have been reviewed by Sielhorst et al. [578] in a literature overview of AR approaches designed for medical displays. After a large gap, Chen et al. [103] published the current state of mixed-reality approaches in the medical domain and also outlined future challenges. In 2020, two survey papers summarized the current trends of VR and AR in medicine and healthcare [11, 89]. The recent movement to understand decision processes in AI, termed explainable AI (XAI), is prominent in many works [623].

2.1 Surface Rendering

The classic baseline technique in surface rendering is indisputably the Marching Cubes algorithm, introduced in 1987 by Lorensen and Cline [385]. Since then, several surface-based techniques with a special focus on medical visualization have appeared. Fang et al. [158] interactively rendered surfaces for medical visualization, suggesting improvements to the original Marching Cubes algorithm. Shieu et al. [574] generated a 3D surface representation and presented its subsequent visualization using Fourier descriptors. Complementary research efforts led to the classification [507] and smoothing [417] of medical surface meshes.

Surface rendering is often applied to display segmented medical image data. The segmented data is typically given as a binary mask, defining whether a voxel belongs to an anatomical structure. Isosurfaces resulting from such binary data exhibit significant staircase artifacts, which attract human attention and distract from the actual properties of the anatomical structures. The artifacts can be severe because medical image data is typically anisotropic with an interslice distance that is much larger than the pixel size within slices. Thus, surface smoothing is a common problem in medical surface visualization.

Surface smoothing algorithms differ in computational effort, resulting in smoothness, and accuracy. Smoothness can be objectively assessed by curvature. Successful smoothing reduces the average curvature of a surface model. Accuracy relates primarily to volume loss, i.e., iterative smoothing may lead to the shrinkage of structures. Bade et al. [28] compared four often used smoothing algorithms with different parameters to derive specific recommendations for different categories of medical surfaces, e.g., compact structures and elongated structures. Among these common techniques is Taubin's LowPass operator that targets high accuracy [612]. *Constrained elastic surface nets* [187] are particularly useful for binary medical surface representations. The advantage of this technique is the restriction of the translation of vertices in the smoothing process to the size of one voxel, i.e., the approach comes with a guarantee for the resulting accuracy.

The smoothing approach by Moench et al. [417] limits the translation of vertices to those that are strongly affected by staircase artifacts (*staircase-aware smoothing*). The same authors also constrained smoothing so that the minimum distances between structures are not affected. A tumor model may be smoothed without compromising the assessment to adjacent risk structures (*distance-aware smoothing*) [418].

Staircase-aware smoothing attracted further attention [662]. Poisson surfaces also turned out to be a viable method for reconstructing smooth medical surfaces [461]. More recently, also learning-based solutions were developed [661]. Furthermore, surface reconstruction workflows for specific structures have been investigated. Such structures comprise the respiratory tract [98, 655], the whole heart [315], and the liver surface [461].

The novel surface model by Pei et al. [469] generates 3D surfaces for organs from volumetric data in a three-stage process. First, they perform organ classification, then apply a modified graph-cut algorithm to segment the entire region of the organ, and finally use geodesic active contours to obtain the surface model. In 2020, Wang et al. [656] visualized 3D surfaces specifically targeting the planning of tumor magnetic inductive thermotherapy.

2.2 Volume Visualization

Volume rendering is a core topic in medical visualization, evidenced by hundreds of publications—among the most influential ones being papers of Karl-Heinz Höhne and colleagues [239, 620]. We identified about 80 publications that address various challenges in visualizing medical volume data. Among the pioneering works in this domain are the approaches by Drebin [143] and Levoy [366] (Fig. 2.3). The essential work from 1986 by Höhne and Bernstein [239] shades 3D images from CT scans using gray-level gradients.

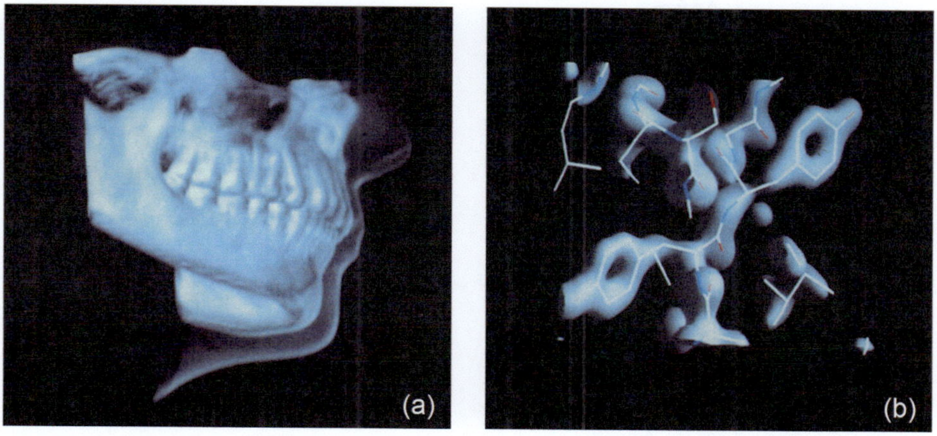

Fig. 2.3 Volume rendering of (a) jaw with semi-transparent skin and (b) ribonuclease from the implementation of Levoy *(©1990 ACM, Reprinted with permission from [366], Figs. 5 and 7)*

The boom in this field begins immediately thereafter, and the following decades see a steady increase in publications.

In the 1990s, many publications established the basic concepts of volume rendering in biomedical visualizations. Kaufman et al. [292] discussed the properties of cell data and the difficulties when rendering them in 3D. Visualization of tomography scans was another important aspect during this time [240, 435]. Tiede et al. [621] defined standards for high-quality rendering of segmented volumetric objects and especially their boundary surfaces. Along with rendering itself, researchers also evaluated display systems for visualizing medical volume data [459]. Performance has been another important aspect of the developed algorithms. Opportunities of parallel processing for real-time volume rendering of medical data were investigated [204, 470]. Shahidi et al. [566] compared surface and volume rendering techniques in medical imaging. Additionally, multimodality [690] and advanced applications of volume visualization in medicine [538] started to play an important role.

The new millennium brought new technologies and new opportunities. Dedicated volume rendering hardware started to be used in rendering systems, such as the VolumePro board [473]. With parallel projection, the system rendered 500 MegaVoxels per second. Its extension (VolumePro 1000) doubled the performance and provided perspective projection to support virtual endoscopy. Engel et al. [150] combined local desktop computers and remote high-end graphics hardware to maximally exploit the visualization capabilities for displaying tomographic data. Increased rendering capabilities introduced more details to the visualization [141]. They also allowed researchers to explore visual enhancement techniques, such as ambient occlusion [525] or opacity peeling [508]. During this period, we have also seen a steady increase in releases that leverage the capabilities of the GPU for volume rendering [152, 584]. Shen et al. [572] designed early real-time immersive visualization environments for the exploration of medical volume data.

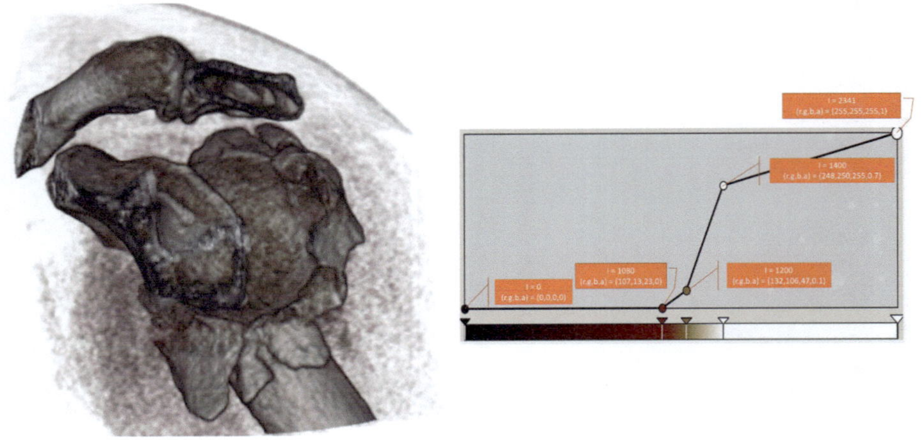

(a) (b)

Fig. 2.4 Volume rendering of a shoulder CT data set (a) and its respective transfer function (b) created in MeVisLab

Since 2010, the research has been directed to enhance visual perception [553, 649]. Yoo et al. [680] investigated similarities in the visual representation of the human body through volumetric datasets and electron microscopy images. Despite the nine orders of magnitude difference in scale, they revealed that the analysis and modeling methods are remarkably similar. Toolkits, such as MeVisLab or VTK (see Fig. 2.4) for visualizing and exploring medical datasets also became widespread [73, 99].

The latest works focus on volume rendering of PET-CT scans [280], volumetric path tracing [394], and perception of semi-transparent structures [151]. An innovative approach was proposed by Stoppel and Bruckner [599], who designed printable tangible wheel cards that can be manipulated to explore parameter settings for volume visualization. Among the latest trends in medical visualization is *cinematic rendering* [128, 149]. The technique involves a novel 3D rendering algorithm to simulate the propagation and interaction of light rays as they pass through the volume data. This approach supports photorealistic rendering, as depicted in Fig. 2.5 showing a comparison to standard volume rendering. Such renderings are currently used in many commercial, FDA-approved products.

Medical visualizations have also been impacted by recent advances in machine learning. In this regard, *Neural Radiance Field* (NeRF) [412] appears as a promising deep-learning technique. The technique reconstructs a volumetric scene as a continuous function from a sparse set of input images. The resulting function can then be rendered using traditional volume rendering approaches, enabling the synthesis of new views. Recently, Maas et al. [389] have shown the use of NeRF for 3D reconstruction from X-ray angiography. Kerbl et al. [295] combined the ideas of NeRF with splatting, a technique traditionally used for continuous

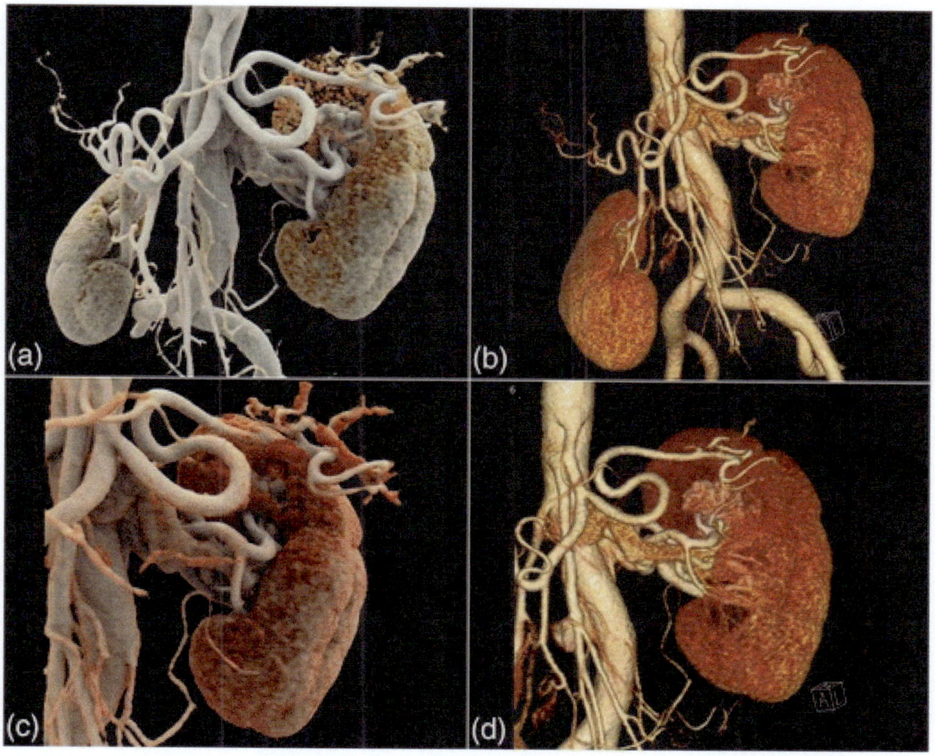

Fig. 2.5 (a), (c) Cinematic rendering of contrast-enhanced 3D CT images of an arteriovenous malformation in the kidney compared to traditional volume rendering (b), (d) [128]. *Image distributed under the terms of the* Creative Commons CC BY 4.0 *license*

image synthesis from point clouds. In their work, the reconstructed scene is represented with 3D Gaussians, which enables significant performance improvements.

2.3 Transfer Functions

Transfer functions (TFs) define the appearance of volume data. They typically map intensity values to brightness and opacity, thus specifying which portions of the data are visible and which contrasts arise. TFs have been extensively studied in both general volume rendering and medical contexts [22, 382]. Over the years, several TF designs have been proposed—some of them with more specific target data in mind. For example, Honigmann et al. [249] suggested an automatic setup of the opacity TF for sonographic data. The automated design of TFs was furthered by Nguyen et al. [436]. Cai et al. [93] enhanced important structures, which are difficult to capture using traditional TF approaches. The underlying algorithm learns a set of rules that can distinguish user-specified target tissues. Ljung et al. [383] utilized TFs as a guide for decompressing the data, as parts of the volume can be represented at low resolution while retaining overall visual quality. Another well-researched area is the design of texture-based TFs. Here, the properties of the texture in the local neighborhood of each voxel are first extracted. The texture descriptor is then used instead of intensity for TF definition. Selver [564] investigated this approach for direct volume rendering of abdominal organs.

Conventional 1D TFs are facing problems to discriminate between tissues with similar intensity values. One of the simplest solutions, proposed by Kniss et al. [306], employs the gradient magnitude as a second dimension. There are also other multi-dimensional approaches. For instance, the size-based TF of Correa and Ma [116] maps the local scale of features in the volume data to color and opacity. In this way, they enable to emphasize features of a certain size. Curvature-based TFs [234] selectively highlight regions with strong changes, e.g., at the boundary of tissues. Distance-based TFs [610] constitute an ideal solution for tasks of exploring the neighborhood of a given structure. They employ the distance to a target, e.g., a tumor or another pathology, to highlight structures in the surroundings. All these methods enable better discrimination of tissue types with similar intensity values than 1D TFs. However, interaction is complex with 2D TFs and radiological workstations do not use them so far.

2.4 Illustrative and Abstracted Representations

In biology and medicine, researchers often deal with dense and complex scenes consisting of many objects in mutually close proximity. Many times, a traditional realistic rendering does not lead to a comprehensive display of the dataset and all its components. Therefore, researchers designed various illustrative and abstract representations to enhance perception and ease the visual communication of the data. In molecular visualization, a typical example is the application of ambient occlusion to 3D atomistic representations of molecules [611]. This significantly improves the perception of cavities and protrusions on the molecular surface. More examples of such methods and techniques can be found in a survey by Kozlíková et al. [320]. In the medical domain, we also evidenced several methods to enhance depth perception [408, 553, 604]. Volumetric halos are a notable example, where an interactively defined halo TF facilitates the perception of occlusions [81].

Visibility enhancements have also been investigated. For example, *smart visibility* is an outstanding concept to control the visibility of structures, such as a tumor in the context of surrounding organs. The depiction of occluding regions is modified, either by removing them (e.g., with *cutaway views*) or by rendering them transparently (e.g., with *ghosted views*). Viola and Gröller [646] introduced smart visibility along with examples from medical volume rendering. Kubisch et al. [332] discussed variants of rendering, e.g., the specific shapes of cut regions and shading, and the application to tumor surgery.

Smart visibility techniques are sometimes referred to as *high-level illustrative techniques*. *Low-level illustrative techniques* deal with the actual rendering styles and comprise silhouette rendering, hatching, and stippling, i.e., classic illustrative techniques known from textbooks in biology and medicine for centuries. While point- and line-based techniques may convey essential shape features, such as major curvature lines, they are usually not sufficient. Two-level volume rendering [221] is an essential concept to combine different rendering styles on a per-object basis. Thus, illustrative techniques and direct volume rendering can be combined.

Tietjen et al. [622] described a concept for the integration of volume, surface, and silhouette rendering (Fig. 2.6). Silhouettes emphasize boundaries and further shape cues can be conveyed with hatching [353] and stippling [29, 197]. While most illustration techniques have been applied to surface data, illustrative volume rendering has also been investigated. An essential example of this line of research is the paper by Bruckner and Gröller [82] on style transfer functions. Other techniques applied to medical volume visualization include surface hatching [142] or silhouettes [546]. Special illustrative techniques have been developed for DTI fiber tracts [606] and vessel visualization [352, 519], for molecular structures [351, 634] and blood flow [67, 635].

Several works adjust techniques from information visualization to the biomedical domain—especially with the advent of visual analytics in medicine and healthcare. For example, Ponciano et al. [481] built a graph-based hierarchy from pre-segmented volume data, which is then used for interactive exploration of the volume. Similarly, Tory et al. [625] utilized parallel coordinates to build an interface for exploratory visualization of volume data. 2D histograms are another option to explore 3D medical data, as proposed by Wesarg and

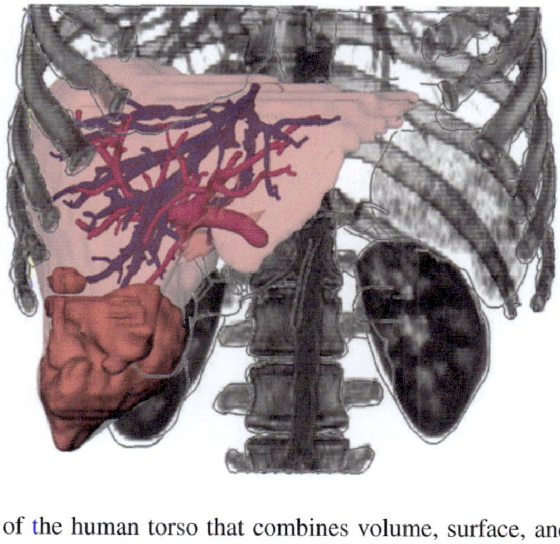

Fig. 2.6 A rendering of the human torso that combines volume, surface, and silhouette rendering by Tietjen et al. [622]. *© 2005 The Author(s), Eurographics Proceedings © 2005 The Eurographics Association. Reproduced by kind permission of the Eurographics Association*

Kirschner [667]. Another notable example is the use of Circos [330] for the representation of omics data. Abstracted views inspired by information visualization were also proposed for the exploration of the Circle of Willis [411].

A number of pioneering works experimented with techniques distorting the original shape of the data to provide an overview and ease their exploration. Multiple reformation approaches can be found in the area of vascular visualizations (Sect. 3.6.4), where the Curved Planar Reformation (CPR) [287] is a notable example. Another exemplary case is the virtual unfolding of a colon. Vilanova and Gröller [644] presented a technique that artificially cut and flattened the colon's tubular and folded shape. Zeng et al. [682] applied harmonic differentials to colon unfolding. Miao et al. [410] developed an approach for creating 2D placenta maps from MRI images. Flattening and reformation of complex three-dimensional shapes were also applied in molecular visualization (Sect. 3.4.3). For example, Halladjian et al. [210] gradually unfolded the complex genome structure into smaller and smaller organizational units.

2.5 Virtual and Augmented Reality in Medicine

In recent years, the accessibility and advancement in devices that support extended reality, such as virtual reality glasses, prompted the development of numerous solutions targeting their use in medical contexts. Therefore, in this section, we discuss the basics of virtual and augmented reality approaches.

2.5.1 Virtual Reality in Medicine

Virtual reality (VR) typically involves the use of glasses, also referred to as head-mounted display (HMD), that enable a stereoscopic visual perception in rather high spatial resolution, a very fast update of a virtual environment in real-time when users rotate their heads (*head tracking*), and the use of controllers that enable the selection of objects, grasping or other kind of virtual object manipulation. Users are fully immersed and have the illusion that they are somewhere else, e.g., in an operating room or in another part of a hospital (Fig. 2.7). The user's movements are tracked and enable navigation in the virtual environment, e.g., a medical student can virtually walk around a patient, initiate some tests, and train an intervention.

The set of affordable VR glasses, such as the HTC Vive, introduced in 2014 makes this illusion possible and VR applications feasible. The field of view (FOV) of VR glasses is ideally the same as the FOV of the human eye. The spatial resolution and the contrast are ideally also high enough to fully exploit our visual perception capabilities. Although the technical development has not yet reached this stage, successful applications in medical treatment and medical training are already possible.

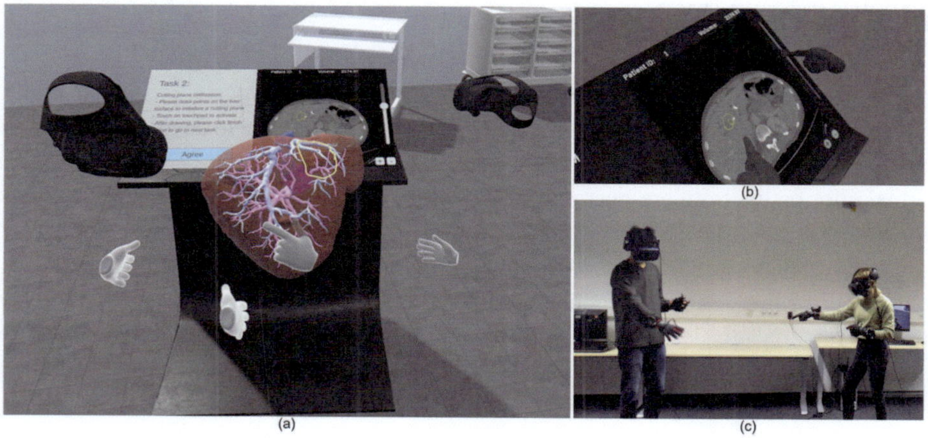

Fig. 2.7 Overview of (a) a collaborative VR prototype for liver surgery planning, where (b) the exploration of 2D slices and tumor contours is possible, similar to (c) the real world *(©2021 IEEE, Reprinted with permission from: [105])*

While VR is focused on visual perception, auditory perception and haptics may be integrated which is potentially valuable for medical applications, such as surgery training, where sound may indicate that instruments reach a critical region and tactile perception may improve the handling of human tissue.

The successful use of VR in such applications requires rather realistic virtual environments that induce a *place illusion* where people literally forget that they are in a computer lab but behave as if they would be somewhere else. Thus, patients feel as if they would be on top of a house to struggle and finally overcome their fear of heights. The "sense of presence" characterizes to what extent this illusion actually exists.

The use of VR in medicine started early with a focus on treating anxieties, such as acrophobia (fear of heights) [530]. VR-based treatment is also available for treating acute and chronic pain and for rehabilitation after a stroke [488]. These approaches are discussed in more detail in Sect. 3.10. Another driving application is surgery training (Sect. 3.9.1), particularly for minimally invasive surgery where the difficult eye-hand coordination and the handling of (long) instruments operating through narrow spaces need to be trained [35].

More recently, the use of VR in medicine has extended to applications where cooperation is essential, e.g., between two surgeons or surgeons and other physicians [106]. Such systems enable also the training of communication skills that are essential in many medical treatment scenarios, such as tumor board discussions, radiological interventions, and surgery.

2.5.2 Augmented Reality in Medicine

Being fully immersed in VR is beneficial for training and some types of medical treatment. However, it means that users do not recognize the reality around them anymore. For surgery (Sect. 3.8), it is desirable, that the real information from an operating room (OR) and the virtual information from pre-operative planning can be combined. This is the major goal of *augmented reality* (AR).

The overlay of virtually generated information on top of live data from an OR is challenging. It requires correctly aligning pre-operative data with the live data. This alignment involves rotation, translation, and scaling of pre-operative data. Typically, a global transform (called *rigid registration*) is not sufficient since the live data includes soft-tissue components, such as deformable organs. Thus, a computationally intense non-rigid registration is required where for different parts of a volume dataset, different transformations are computed.

Examples of medical AR include displaying the boundaries of a tumor (from a 3D model) on top of an organ during surgery to guide the surgeons. Also, essential vascular structures may be shown on top of an organ before the surgeon cuts. Clearly, there are high demands for the accuracy and reliability of the displayed information—the position where tumors and vessels are shown must be correct. A taxonomy of augmented and mixed-reality approaches for image-guided surgery was presented by Kersten-Oertel et al. [297].

Also, AR requires appropriate hardware in particular AR glasses. Like VR headsets they are tracked, making it possible to record their position and orientation. Reliable tracking is a prerequisite for a correct display of the aligned virtual information. The Microsoft HoloLens is a popular type of AR glasses that is also used for a lot of medical applications [223, 438]. However, there are also special AR glasses developed for use in an operating room.

2.6 Available Software in BioMedical Visualization

In this section, we discuss currently available software in the domain of Biological and Medical Visualization. It is worth noting that while we aim to provide an informative overview, the compilation discussed below may not be exhaustive. It focuses on well established and primarily freely available software and draws upon the prior insights and experiences of the co-authors. A more comprehensive list of the software is available at our accompanying website: https://biomedvis-book.fi.muni.cz/.

Software in BioVis Research. The evolution of software tools in the BioVis domain has been rich and diverse. Here we list examples of (epi)genome browsers, visual analytic tools for single-cell —omics data, network visualization, and general-purpose molecular visualization. Since the nature of research in this area often necessitates integration with scripting environments, we also remark on notable visualization libraries and packages.

- Integrative Genomics Viewer (IGV): IGV is a high-performance browser for the exploration of various types of 1D sequencing data. The tool is open source and available as desktop and web applications. Furthermore, it is also available as a JavaScript library and Python package, allowing easy integration in computational notebooks.
- WashU Epigenome Browser: It is a web-based tool consisting of several visual components aiding the exploration of complex epigenomic datasets. It integrates multiple configurable views including 1D data tracks, 2D contact maps, image data, and 3D structure view.
- Gosling: Gosling presents a grammar-based toolkit for interactive and scalable genomics data visualization offering various 1D and 2D views. It enables the users to explore and transition between different scales in the datasets. It is available as a JavaScript library and Python package.
- Loupe Browser: 10X Genomics' Loupe Browser is an example of many browsing tools for high-dimensional single-cell genomics data provided by a manufacturer of the corresponding data acquisition machines. It focuses on annotations of these data through dimensionality reduction and filtering. Similar tools include Cytobank or CELLxGENE.
- Cytosplore: Cytosplore is a desktop visual analytics tool targeted at the analysis of single-cell proteomics data. It integrates dimensionality reduction, clustering, and interactive visualization of results. This provides direct feedback on analysis results and supports steering of analysis algorithms.
- Vitessce: Vitessce provides scalable, linked visualizations that support the visual analysis of spatial (and non-spatial) cellular and molecular observations. It is an open-source framework, providing a web app, as well as python and R integrations.
- Seurat: Seurat is an R package designed for the exploration of single-cell RNA-sequencing data. Seurat enables users to identify and interpret sources of heterogeneity from single-cell transcriptomic measurements and to integrate diverse types of single-cell data. It provides a scripting-based interface in R. A similar package for the Python language is Scanpy.
- Cytoscape: Cytoscape is nowadays a comprehensive, extensible framework for the visualization and visual analysis of large networks. This includes a vast array of tools targeted at biological networks and pathways. Many of them link back to Cytoscape's roots as a visualization software environment for biomolecular interaction networks.
- UCSF ChimeraX: This tool for molecular visualization provides users with a wide range of functions for interactive exploration and manipulation with molecular structures. It is freely available for nonprofit and personal use.
- PyMOL: It is one of the most widely used and robust open-source tools for molecular visualization, which offers to view, share, and analyze molecular datasets. The users can also create animations and movies, and generate high-quality images for publications.
- Mol*: To increase the accessibility, the authors of Mol* aimed to create a web-based open-source toolkit for visualization and analysis of large-scale molecular data. Optimizations

in rendering and data handling enable the users to simultaneously visualize hundreds of structures, play animations, and display cell-level models.

- Jmol/JSMol: The web-based package JSmol (and its standalone version Jmol) is another open-source molecular viewer. The main benefit of JSmol is that it can be simply embedded into other web pages.
- VMD: Visual Molecular Dynamics (VMD) is a molecular visualization program that focuses on displaying, animating, and analyzing large biomolecular systems. It allows the users built-in scripting to introduce customized functions. VMD is multiplatform and open source, and has a very large user base.
- MegaMol: This system was originally created as a prototyping framework for the development of new visualization approaches and rendering algorithms in molecular visualization. It still serves as a tool for developers but also provides the users with a robust base of available functions.
- UnityMol: UnityMol is another prototyping platform implemented in the Unity3D game engine. This opens new possibilities for developers and users, as it also offers the virtual reality version of UnityMol. It is open source, with a free license for academics.
- Molecular Maya: This free plug-in for Autodesk Maya is a very good solution for those who want to import, model, and animate molecular structures in a 3D modeling environment. It serves both scientists and artists to generate high-quality animations of molecular mechanisms.
- BioRender: This simple drag-and-drop online tool enables the users to quickly sketch illustrations of molecular structures and other phenomena. It is very suitable for generating schematic images from a set of predefined objects. BioRender provides users with a large library of scientifically accurate and high-resolution images of objects to start with. The tool is freely available for personal use.

Software in MedVis Research. Among the tools available for the visualization of medical data, we focus on those that stand out for their flexibility, community support, and varied applications. We also include versatile general-purpose scientific visualization tools.

- 3D Slicer: A free and open-source platform, 3D Slicer excels in medical image analysis and visualization. It offers a wide range of functionalities, including segmentation, registration, and visualization of MRI, CT, and PET scans. Its extensive community support ensures regular updates and a vast repository of modules catering to diverse research needs.
- MeVisLab: Primarily used in medical imaging research, MeVisLab provides a comprehensive environment for developing image processing and rendering algorithms. While it is free for non-commercial use, commercial licenses are available for enterprise applications. The framework's strength lies in its modular architecture, facilitating rapid prototyping and integration of custom algorithms.

- MITK: The Medical Imaging Interaction Toolkit (MITK) offers a platform for the development of interactive medical image processing software. It is open source and supported by a large community. Its features include 3D visualization, image segmentation, and image registration, making it a valuable tool in medical research and clinical practice.
- Inviwo: Known for its focus on interactive data visualization, Inviwo provides a versatile environment for scientific computing and visualization. It is not specifically tailored for medical visualization. Its flexibility, however, allows researchers to adapt it to various domains (such as cell imaging and histopathological slices). Inviwo is open source and supported by an active community.
- ParaView: Widely used in scientific computing and visualization, ParaView offers powerful tools for analyzing large datasets. While it is not specifically designed for medical visualization, it has been utilized in medical research for tasks like fluid dynamics simulation and computational modeling. ParaView is open source and benefits from extensive community support and contributions.
- VTK and ITK: The Visualization Toolkit (VTK) and the Insight Segmentation and Registration Toolkit (ITK) were both developed by Kitware. VTK focuses on 3D computer graphics and visualization, while ITK specializes in image processing. Both are open source and widely used in medical imaging research and clinical applications.

Application Fields

3

In this chapter, we discuss the research trends within individual application fields according to our taxonomy. Including all papers identified within our literature survey would not be feasible, and we, therefore, focus on the most influential works. The entire literature corpus and its categorization can be accessed and explored at our searchable repository at biomedvis-book.fi.muni.cz. Each of the following sections discusses the most prominent literature in the given application field, ordered by the scale in which they act. Within each subsection, we will comment on the trends and evolution thereof, with regard to the other dimensions—namely the data, stakeholders, tasks, and scale of application. We indicate the most influential authors with capitalization.

3.1 Omics

The term *—omics* loosely comprises a number of methods, primarily in systems biology that end in the suffix *omics*, such as *genomics*, *transcriptomics*, *proteomics*, or *metabolomics*. Generally, these methods produce quantitative data on the structure, function, and dynamics of biological organisms. We will first focus on functional properties, while further aspects are discussed in later sections. For example, structural genomics models protein structures by analyzing the genome. In this respect, methods for the spatial visualization of proteins are relevant, which are discussed in Sect. 3.4. Connectomics, dealing with mapping connections in the brain are discussed in Sect. 3.7.

Omics data acquisition is a new and rapidly evolving area. The first references to —omics data are all from the area of genomics and date back to the late 1980s. Literature using the —omics term is very sparse until around the year 2000. In Fig. 3.1 we see initial visualization approaches appearing in the 1990s. The early works are mostly con-

K. Furmanová et al., *BioMedical Visualization*, Synthesis Lectures on Visualization,
https://doi.org/10.1007/978-3-031-66789-3_3

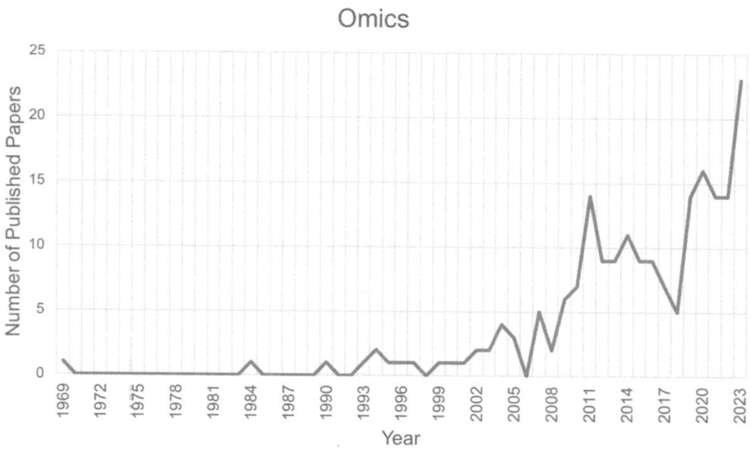

Fig. 3.1 Number of *omics visualization* papers published over time

cerned with depicting *genomic sequences* [675] and particularly comparative visualizations for finding similar patterns over multiple aligned sequences [107, 108]. These works represent sequences either as a line chart or as a series of letters. Letters represent different structures, such as *nucleotide bases* or *amino acids* [218, 552]. In 2001, the Human Genome Project published a draft sequencing of the human *genome* [345, 641]. This initiated a steep growth in novel —omics data acquisition methods and subsequently corresponding visualization methods and tools. A good tool-focused overview of earlier work has been presented in a 2010 special issue of Nature Methods on biological data visualization [154].

3.1.1 Genomic Sequence Visualization

Depicting the genome is a core area in —omics visualization. The genome contains the entire genetic information of an organism and can be described on multiple scales. Very simplified, on the highest scale, the genome is described by a set of *chromosomes*. A chromosome is a long strand of *DNA* (deoxyribonucleic acid) coiled up into the iconic double helix. The DNA double helix consists of a sequence of *nucleotides* bound into pairs on the two strands, which are coiled together. The nucleotides are typically identified by a single letter corresponding to their base, i.e., either one of **A**denine, **T**hymine, **C**ytosine, or **G**uanine. As each nucleotide can only bind to one other nucleotide, the two strands are complementary and we also speak of base pairs instead of a singular base. In clinical practice, genome analysis is used for example for identifying rare disorders or prenatal aneuploidy screening that involves the identification of extra or missing chromosomes in unborns.

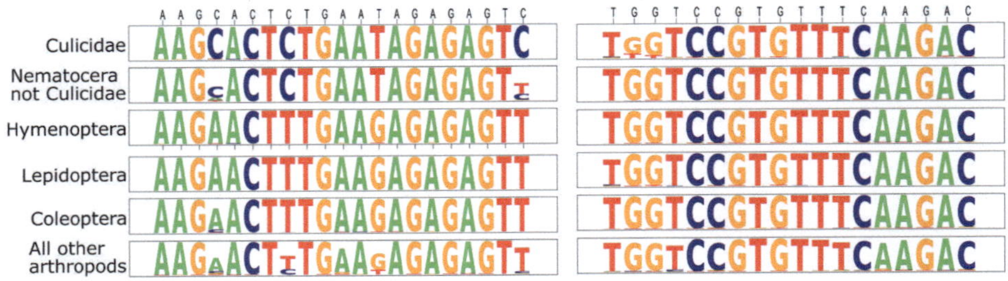

Fig. 3.2 Examples of sequence logos for different species of insects [468]. *Image distributed under the terms of the* Creative Commons CC BY 4.0 *license*

The visualization of genomic data is subdivided into two areas:

- *Abstract genome sequence data* is commonly visualized using standard information visualization techniques.
- *Geometric models of the genome* are visualized with computer graphics-based rendering techniques. These are closely related to the methods described in Sect. 3.4.

Nielsen et al. [439] provide a tool-focused overview of genome visualization techniques. More recently, Nusrat et al. [446] survey tasks, techniques, and tools for visualizing genomic sequences and provide taxonomies for all three aspects. Genomic sequences are long series of a single qualitative attribute. A number of visualization techniques lend themselves to this type of data. A straightforward way is to print the corresponding sequence of letters, for comparison purposes introduced as sequence logos [552] (Fig. 3.2). Until now this is an iconic representation for genomic sequences. Mauve [129] introduced the use of vertical lines with different color hues to represent class information.

A major challenge in visualizing sequence data is the extreme size of the sequences, e.g., approximately three billion base pairs for the human genome. Wong et al. [671] proposed the use of space-filling curves to efficiently map whole bacterial genome sequences to 2D screens. They layout pixels with four color hues, each according to one base letter, in a 2D grid using different space-filling curves. The concept was later picked up by Gu et al. [202]. Ngyen et al. [437] presented a spiral representation to fit long one-dimensional sequences on 2D displays. Even though these methods use the given space more efficiently, they are hard to read and thus have rarely been used.

A common way to tackle the large scale of the data is aggregation. The complete sequence can be aggregated by dividing it into regular-sized blocks and summarizing the corresponding sub-sequences [117], often providing full detail with additional (in-place) views or Focus+Context methods. Alternatively, data-driven aggregation is possible, e.g., by identifying repeating short sub-sequences, which are then represented in different ways. In ABySS-Explorer [440], Nielsen et al. map short sub-sequences to glyph-based representations, which they combine into longer assemblies in a graph. Spell et al. [595] as well as O'Brien et al. [447] identify repeating sub-sequences and highlight them by connection, using arcs on top of the 1D sequence plot. Their method can be used on the complete sequence without aggregation. They also present a visual aggregation of the identified sub-sequences.

While the majority of methods for sequence analysis target 2D displays, there are a few works in 3D. Thiagarajan and Gao [618] align letter-based sequences in 2D and use the third dimension to visualize the support for their alignment. They target 2D computer screens, but similar methods have been presented also for virtual reality systems [4, 289, 523].

3.1.2 Comparative Visualization and Sequence Alignment

A major application for sequencing data is a comparison between species and subspecies, such as strains of bacteria (*pan-genomes*), for example, to form hypotheses on the function of genes. To compare multiple sequences, highly similar matching sub-sequences, which are known as *orthologs*, are calculated and used to highlight similar areas or to align sequences. An overview of tools for the visualization of multiple alignments is provided by Procter et al. [494]. Set-based information, such as the overlap of contained sub-sequences over multiple sequences, has traditionally been visualized using Venn diagrams [133, 613] (e.g., Fig. 3.3a) but is slowly replaced by UpSet [368]. UpSet combines bar charts, indicating the frequency of classes, and an explicit representation of overlaps between classes using connected dots (see Fig. 3.3b). For a detailed analysis, the 1D visual representations for abstract sequence depictions as presented above are commonly used in comparative approaches. Here multiple sequences are shown as rows in a grid [570, 575]. Aggregation of sub-sequences across multiple sequences and representation as blocks is commonly employed to ease comparison [13, 261, 580]. In elaborate methods, the sizes of these blocks typically result from a data-driven definition. Multiple sequences are aligned and laid out on-screen based on the agreement between the sequences, rather than aligning them with the edge of the viewport [25, 231].

Beyond showing multiple sequences as individual rows, a number of more explicit approaches for comparison have been introduced. Kultys et al. [334] and Sakai and Aerts [536] concurrently introduced a line representation, where the horizontal axis corresponds to the sequence and the vertical axis to the different classes. Multiple sequences are then represented as lines and bundled for comparison. Icelogo [110] extends the common letter sequences by aligning and aggregating sequences, reducing them to only significant matches, and scaling or coloring letters by frequency. Pan-Tetris [225] explicitly encodes differences over multiple genomic sequences as colored arrow glyphs.

Synteny analysis aims at comparing blocks of sub-sequences to derive preservation of such blocks within two compared sets of chromosomes, for example, from different species. Cinteny [581] uses (stacked) bar charts to represent the chromosomes. For a source genome, each chromosome is represented as a solid colored bar. For the comparand, orthologs with respect to the base genome are colored according to the color of the corresponding

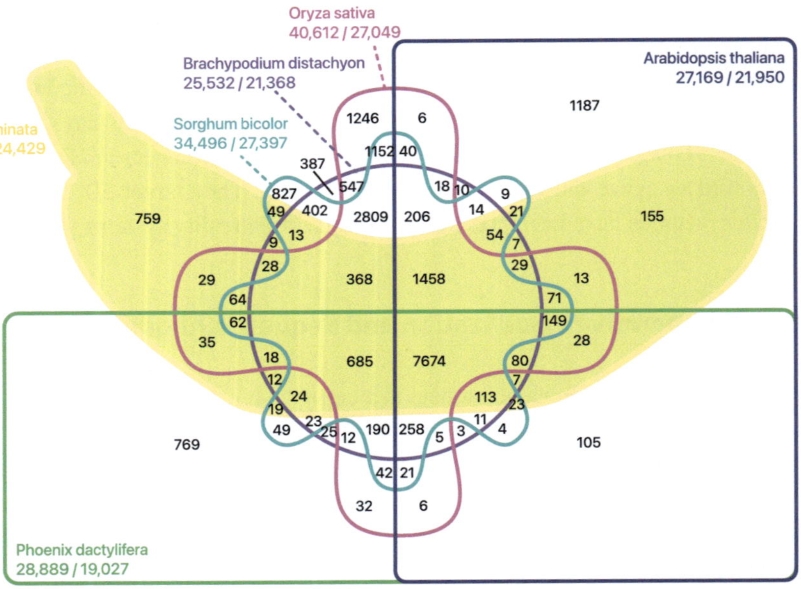

(a)

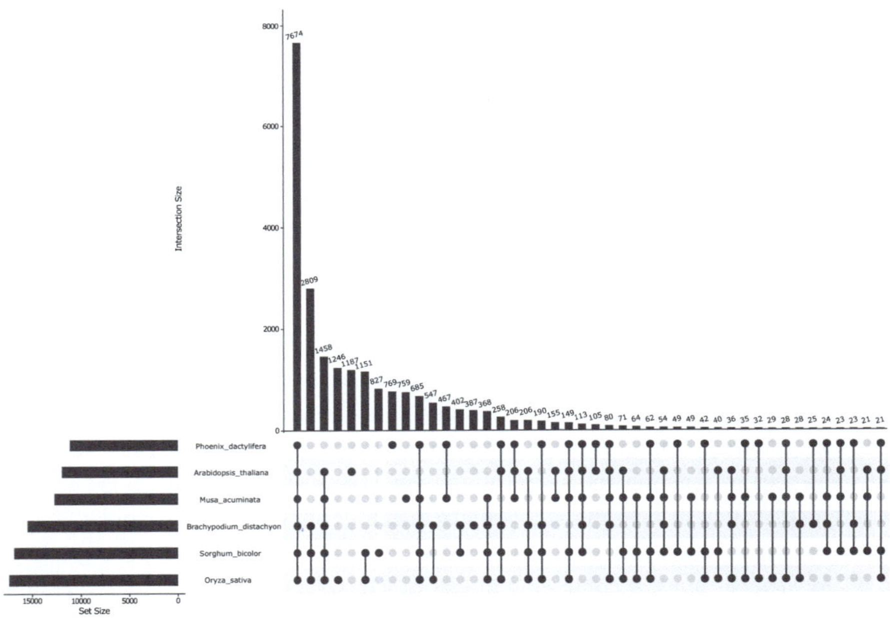

(b)

Fig. 3.3 Comparison of the banana genome with other species, visualized as (a) Venn diagram (recreated after [133]) and using (b) Upset [368]. The UpSet app is available at https://upset.app. *Images distributed under the terms of the* Creative Commons CC BY 4.0 *license*

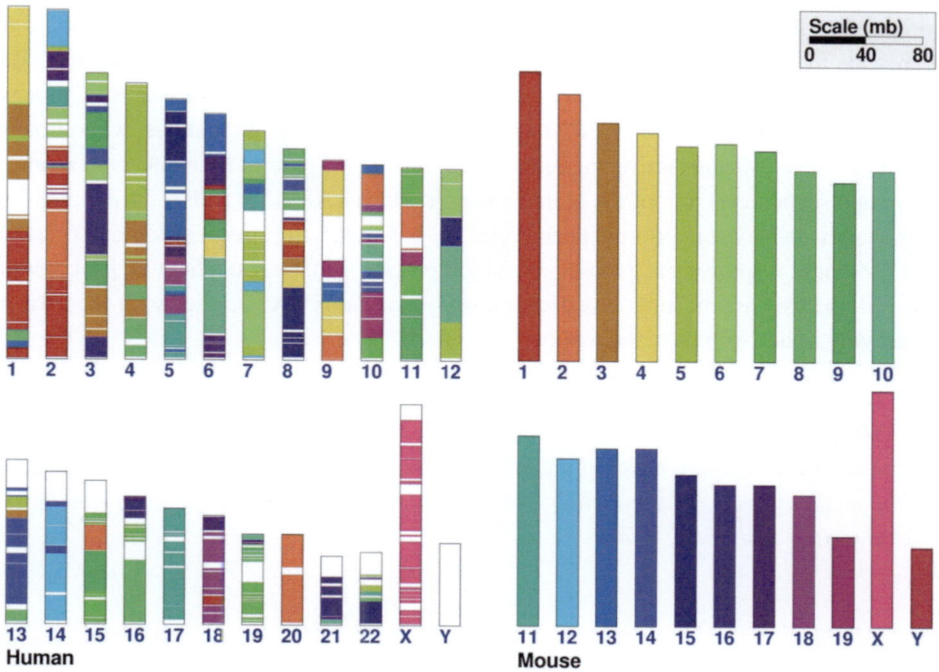

Fig. 3.4 Comparison of the mouse (source) and human (comparand) genome using Cinteny [581]. *Image distributed under the terms of the* Creative Commons CC BY 4.0 *license*

chromosome (Fig. 3.4). Synteny Explorer [85] extends this concept in several ways to improve the identification of orthologs, for example, by connection or animation. Mizbee [407] allows multiscale synteny comparison. In the main view, chromosomes are laid out in a circular fashion, and orthologs of a selected chromosome of interest are highlighted by connection.

3.1.3 Genome Wide Association Studies

Special cases of comparative sequence analysis are *Genome Wide Association Studies* (GWAS). GWAS are large-scale studies, capturing and comparing the genome of many individuals, with the goal of finding associations between genetic variants and diseases or non-disease traits (e.g., height) of those individuals through statistical associations. Statistical analysis of such associations is out of the scope of this work, but the resulting associations are commonly visualized.

The standard visualizations for GWAS results are Manhattan plots, likely introduced by Kammerer et al. [283] in 2004, and subsequently named after their resemblance to a dense city skyline. Manhattan plots are essentially scatterplots, where each dot represents a genetic variant. The horizontal axis is used for the position in the genome, and the vertical axis represents the significance of the association with the corresponding trait of interest. The main change from the original plot is the introduction of interactive versions. LocusTrack [126] combines the standard Manhattan plot with annotation features, while LocusZoom [495] enables interactive zooming. Grace et al. [199] present Manhattan++, an interactive and scalable version of the Manhattan plot. PheGWAS [182] adds a third dimension for comparison between different phenotypes and represents the effect sizes as a 3D surface or a 2D height map over the genome × phenotype axes. Finally, Aupetit et al. [24] present a visual analysis approach to investigate kinship data in GWAS studies with the goal of identifying issues with the data quality.

> *Omics sequence visualization presented in Sect.* 3.1 *generally deals with* ***static and high-dimensional abstract data.*** *The data are acquired on the* ***molecular scale.*** *The methods are mostly targeting* ***clinical researchers,*** *and they support primarily* ***exploration and analysis tasks.***

3.2 Interaction Networks and Pathways

Beyond individual sequences, systems biology is concerned with the (pairwise) interaction of biological entities, such as *protein–protein interaction* or *metabolic interactions*, as well as complete sequences of interactions, referred to as *pathways*. Such information is typically represented as networks, where nodes correspond to the entities, and entities that interact are connected by a link. In Fig. 3.5, we see that this topic attracted the attention of visualization research in the 2000s when numerous tools, such as Cytoscape [568] appeared, followed by a peak and subsequent decline in the number of publications in the 2010s.

Interaction Networks. Gehlenborg et al. [181] present a number of tools to visualize interaction networks. Standard graph layout techniques, including node-link diagrams [71, 235] and matrix visualizations [434] are commonly used to visualize these data. As of today, Cytoscape [568] has established itself as the standard tool for visualization of biological networks. A main factor for its success is the modular architecture, which allows for the creation of custom plug-ins. Many recent developments have been contributed in this way by the large community. Droste et al. [145] present a system to create easily customizable visualizations of biochemical networks using node-link diagrams. They propose a system with different abstraction levels and combine it with customizable styles for different types of biochemical networks. This allows users to focus on the structure of the network. The assignment of visual properties can then be done using styles for the specific type of network.

A challenge for visualizing interaction networks is their scale with thousands of items and interactions [181]. Most discussed works rely on a manual placement in the node-link diagrams, which is infeasible for the scales at hand. More recent approaches use

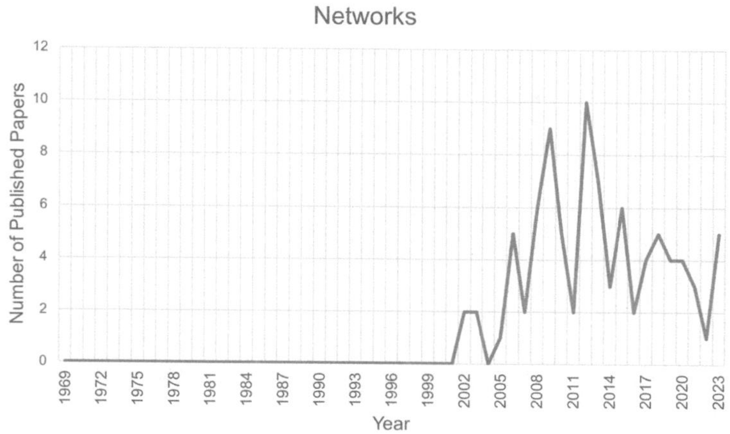

Fig. 3.5 Number of *interaction networks and pathways visualization* papers published over time

force-directed layouts [668]. Schreiber et al. [554] presented a system that can produce automatic layouts in different styles, including force-directed ones, following the conventions for different kinds of biological networks. Dinkla et al. [140] tackle the scale issue in matrix visualizations by exploiting the sparsity of gene regulatory networks. They split networks into weakly connected blocks, which are concatenated into a cascading layout.

A common task in exploring biological networks is the identification and exploration of *motifs*, small connected sub-graphs that occur frequently. MAVisto [555] combines automatic detection of such motifs with a node-link visualization of the network as well as other information in a visual analysis tool. Kavosh [290] and visGReMLIN [509] extend this work, providing more sophisticated motif extraction algorithms, scaling to larger networks and motifs.

Pathways. A biological pathway describes a series of interactions that lead to a product such as a specific chemical molecule. For typical analysis tasks, several pathways are combined into a larger combined network. Matrix views are not suitable for these types of networks, as typically the interactions are traced over several steps. A pathway also has a direction in which the chemical reaction occurs that needs to be visualized. Traditionally, the layout for such networks is painstakingly handcrafted on large-scale posters and the results have been used in educating generations of biology students. As such, it is important that interactive visualizations respect these layouts when adding functionality. Lambert et al. [344] abstract five constraints from this requirement: *closeness* to the original pathway information, node *duplication* avoidance, *topology* preservation, pseudo-orthogonal *edge drawing*, and minimization of *clutter*. They combine automatic node placement and edge bundling to create pathway-preserving layouts of metabolic networks. Wu et al. [676] introduce automatic layouting for pathway networks using an urban planning metaphor. They impose a

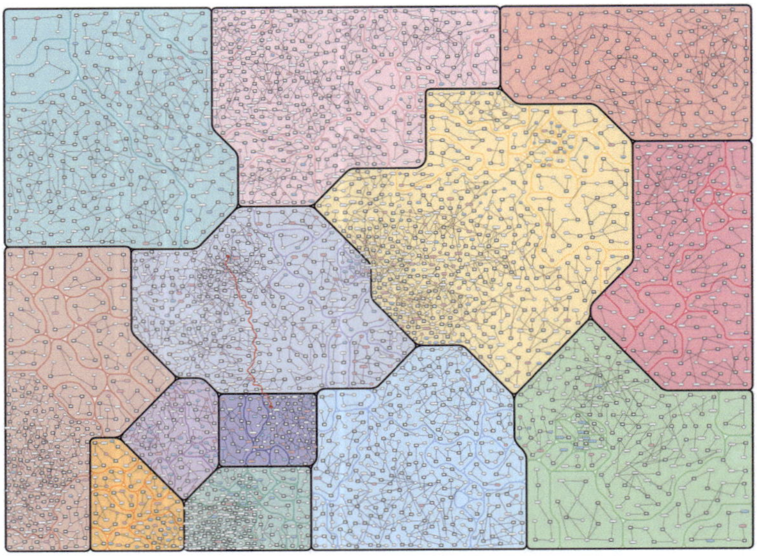

Fig. 3.6 Redrawing the human metabolic pathway map from KEGG [285] with the technique proposed by Wu et al. [677]. *Image courtesy of Hsiang-Yun Wu, St. Pölten University of Applied Sciences*

city block-like grid, partitioned into sub-blocks and used to route pathways to maintain the global and local context simultaneously. They also propose a different approach (Fig. 3.6) based on area balancing and hierarchical partitioning of the available space using Voronoi tessellations [677].

Recently, Murray et al. [430] presented a task taxonomy for the analysis of pathway data, including *attribute*, *relationship*, and *modification* tasks. Cerebral [34] enables multivariate analysis and comparison with the attribute-task set. It uses small multiples to show different experimental conditions within a pathway network. An earlier version was also implemented as a Cytoscape plug-in [33]. Fung et al. [166] present a comparison of overlap in biological networks by the juxtaposition of node-link diagrams as well as layering the juxtaposed diagrams in 2.5D. enRoute [465] allows the user interactive extraction of paths from pathway maps. It offers re-layouting of the network with the goal of highlighting the extracted path. MINERVA [179] and Caleydo [601] focus on the modification task. They provide interactive visualization and editing of such networks. MINERVA focuses on easy interaction and annotation tools while Caleydo adds linking and brushing and interactive queries.

The interaction and pathway visualizations presented in Sect. 3.2 generally deal with ***static and high-dimensional abstract data.*** *The data are acquired on the* ***molecular scale.*** *The methods are mostly targeting* ***clinical researchers,*** *and they support primarily* ***exploration and analysis tasks.***

3.3 Gene and Protein Expression

Besides the qualitative analysis of sequences, in the last 15 years, a vast number of quantitative measurements have been introduced into the —omics space. In particular gene and protein *expression*, i.e., the quantity of genes or proteins in a given sample, are nowadays commonly measured and produce large amounts of high-dimensional data. Like in many other areas, visualization research naturally follows the technological advancements in this field. In Fig. 3.7, we see that the first visualization techniques appeared in the 2000s with a first peak in 2008. These methods focus mostly on data of limited size. A tool-focused overview of visualization methods for the early quantitative data is provided by Gehlenborg et al. [181]. Since the late 2010s, we have seen another spike in publications related to the development of new high-throughput techniques and high-resolution imaging techniques posing new challenges for data analysis.

In the early days, the expression of a few, selected genes or proteins was measured typically in *bulk*, i.e., from pieces of tissue describing a region of the analyzed specimen. For these early methods, standard multi-dimensional data visualization methods have been common. Scatterplots and scatterplot matrices (SPLOMs) have been used to depict the expression of two genes or proteins [357, 464, 522]. Parallel coordinate plots (PCPs) have been proposed [36, 137, 357, 600], but are rarely used in the domain. Cvek et al. [127] presented the use of self-organizing maps [313] to derive a one-dimensional organization of expression data. They then use the resulting 1D space as an additional axis in standard scatterplots or Radviz [238] displays. Another very common representation is heatmap [232], directly encoding the data matrix and mapping the expression values to color. Even early data sizes create matrices that are often too large to inspect individual items on a heatmap.

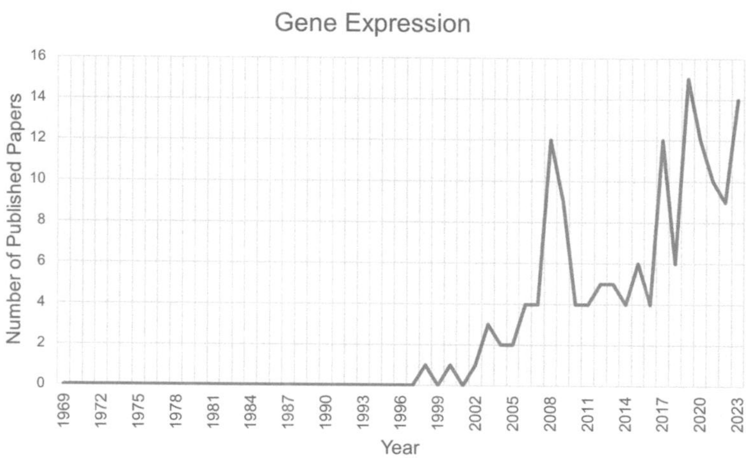

Fig. 3.7 Number of *gene expression visualization* papers published over time

Thus, they are commonly used in combination with clustering and row/column sorting [569], enabling the identification of groups and linked secondary views for detail analysis [36, 540].

Dimensionality Reduction. Modern data acquisition techniques [456] have shifted the focus from bulk to *single-cell*. These methods support the simultaneous measurements of thousands of genes in individual cells at high throughput, producing datasets consisting of matrices with millions of cells/rows and tens of thousands of genes/columns [95, 144, 565, 689]. Especially the large number of dimensions forced a paradigm shift away from the direct representation in SPLOMs or PCPs towards dimensionality reduction (DR). While principal component analysis (PCA) had been used early on for DR [384], the introduction of the non-linear t-distributed stochastic neighbor embedding (t-SNE) [390] to the —omics space [18, 193] started a wave to adapt existing and create new DR methods. Neighborhood-based DR methods like t-SNE preserve local neighborhoods from the original space. Similar items, i.e., cells, will be close together in the embedding space and can easily be identified in the visual representation, which is typically a scatterplot (Fig. 3.8, middle).

A number of optimizations have been introduced to tune t-SNE to single-cell analysis. For example, Belkina et al. [44] present automatic hyper-parameter optimization while Kobak and Berens [307] focus on the initialization of the optimization process. The original t-SNE implementation can only handle a few thousand data points. Given the large number of cells in recent single-cell studies, scalability is important. Linderman et al. [375] present a variant of t-SNE that works in the Fourier domain to reduce complexity.

UMAP [40, 400] is closely related to t-SNE [308], but uses a different optimization, leading to a considerably improved computational performance. Besides computational efficiency, visualizing millions of items in a scatterplot leads to clutter. Van Unen et al. [630]

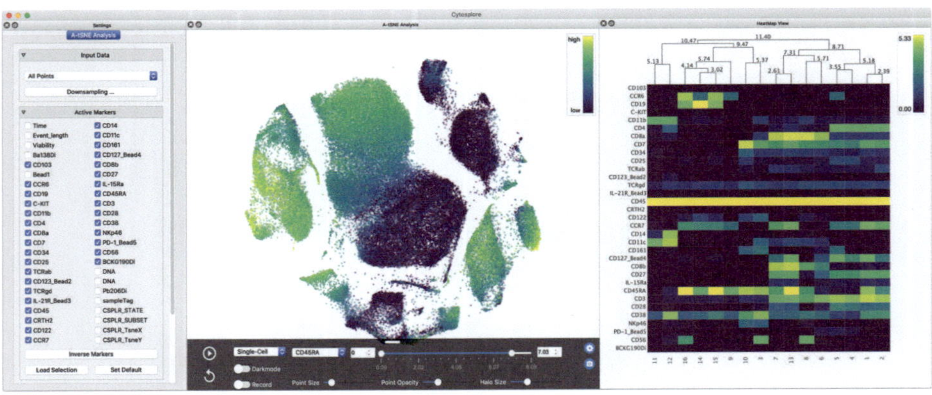

Fig. 3.8 Visualization of a large single-cell dataset using Cytosplore [243]. The middle part shows a t-SNE embedding where each point is a cell. The layout is according to cell similarities, which is based on the expression of different proteins. The expression of one of the proteins is used to color the points. The right side shows the expression (color) of these proteins (rows) for different cell clusters (columns) in a heatmap. *Image created by Thomas Höllt, TU Delft, for this book*

have adapted hierarchical-SNE (HSNE) to single-cell analysis, providing a hierarchical approach with interactive exploration. Later on, CyteGuide [244] introduced guidance for the exploration of these hierarchical embeddings. While t-SNE and UMAP are dominant when it comes to visualizing cell similarities, a number of other DR methods have been presented for this task [393, 648, 679].

Recently, efforts have gone beyond visualization focused on cell similarities and show *cell development* using DR mechanics. PHATE [424], PAGA [670], or Density Path [104], shift the focus from neighborhood preservation in DR to global structures to preserve such information. Wanderlust [47] extracts trajectories from neighborhood graphs in a high-dimensional space and visualizes the related expression profiles over the trajectories with line plots. To scale to large data sizes, multiscale PHATE [333] and PAGA strongly rely on topology-preserving hierarchies introduced with HSNE. Huang et al. [251] present a comparison of relevant DR methods in the —omics field.

Clustering. Aggregating the columns of a data matrix through DR is one option to enable an effective visualization. Alternatively, the items or rows are combined through clustering. For a discussion of general clustering methods in the single-cell field we refer to Liu et al. [381]. Here, we will summarize clustering methods that have a strong visualization aspect. ACCENSE [571] and DensVM [39] are based on t-SNE and cluster the 2D t-SNE embedding using density estimation in the embedding space. SPADE [497] employs hierarchical clustering, while FlowSOM [176] uses self-organizing maps in the original space for the clustering. Both use a minimum spanning tree to visualize the resulting clusters as a node-link diagram. Phenograph [365] and X-shift [539] extract clusters from a neighborhood graph constructed in a high-dimensional space and visualize cluster representatives using t-SNE.

Visual Analytics. While many of the described methods are used for communicating results, they are also employed in exploratory analysis. Consequently, a number of visual analysis and visual analytics approaches include these methods. Cytosplore (Fig. 3.8) introduces an interactive workflow for cell-type identification based on high-dimensional protein expressions. It integrates SPADE clustering with t-SNE and later HSNE [243, 245]. Single Cell Explorer [160], iS-CellR [467], and ASAP [174] implement similar workflows, combining DR with secondary detail views, but for single-cell gene expression data. Brainscope [252] introduces a novel dual t-SNE. This work links embeddings of the original data and the transposed data matrix. Genes are grouped according to their occurrence, to analyze which genes show up in which samples.

Spatial Expression Data. In parallel to expression data, acquired from samples without specific locations, similar data acquisition methods for spatial data have been developed. In early data acquisition methods, the data matrix was essentially extended by the spatial location of the acquired data points, e.g., corresponding to an individual cell. Rübel et al. [532] and Meyer et al. [406] combine the spatial layout of cells in fruit fly embryos with their gene expressions. These early works handle manageable data sizes of a few thousand cells and tens of genes. As such, they directly show the spatial configuration in 3D and unrolled in 2D, respectively. Rübel et al. cluster the cells according to their gene expressions and map the cell clusters to color hues in the spatial layout. Meyer et al. map color to the expression of a selected gene. Both use linked views to show the gene expression in more detail.

More recently, high-resolution imaging techniques such as MERFISH [102] or imaging mass cytometry [188] support the acquisition of *tissue slide* images at sub-cellular resolution. Every pixel contains expression information on tens of proteins to thousands of genes. CellProfiler [275] combines the segmentation of such images with their direct visualization. The visual representation of the high-dimensional gene or protein expression is, however, limited to three dimensions mapped to the red, green, and blue channels of the output image. Facetto [327] and CytoMAP [598] are complete visual analytics systems, including unsupervised cell-type identifications, DR plots for cell-type visualizations, and integrated interactive analysis tools. histoCAT [543] and ImaCytE [591] extend these concepts with the exploration of spatial cell-neighborhood patterns using statistical analyses and visual glyphs, respectively (Fig. 3.9). Somarakis et al. later extend ImaCytE with functionality for comparing cohorts of images based on cell types and spatial organization [589, 590].

> *The most widely used approaches in Sect.* 3.3 *deal with* **static and high-dimensional abstract data,** *but spatial information is becoming more and more relevant. At the same time, expression data is moving from being acquired at* **tissue scale to cell scale**. *The methods are mostly targeting* **clinical researchers,** *and they primarily support* **exploration and analysis tasks.**

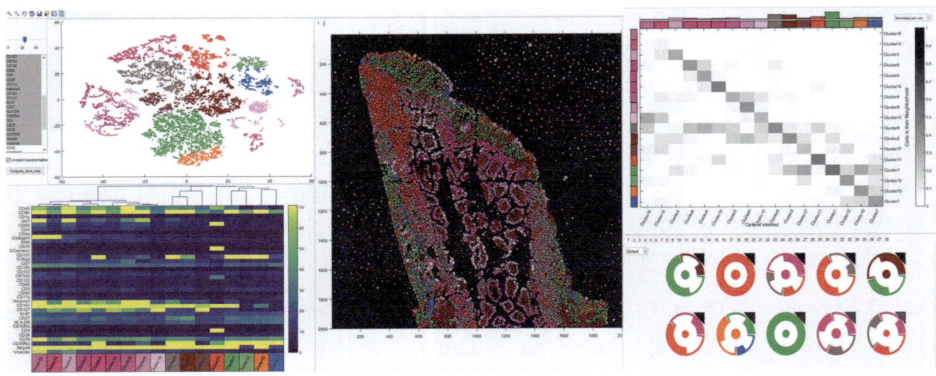

Fig. 3.9 Visual analysis of imaging mass cytometry data using ImaCytE [591]. *Image distributed under the terms of the* Creative Commons CC BY 4.0 *license*

3.4 Visualization of Biological Structures

In this section, we discuss research and techniques developed for the visualization and analysis of biological structures. Here a dominant topic is molecular visualization which has evolved from static representations of small molecules to dynamic representations of crowded cellular environments. An in-depth survey of this topic was published by Kozlíková et al. [320]. As can be seen in Fig. 3.10, visualization of biological structures particularly molecular visualization is one of the oldest branches of visualization altogether. The first approaches appeared in the 1970s, e.g., the molecular-surface representation by Lee and Richards [360]. From the 2000s on we see an uptake in publications which can be related to advances in GPU-based rendering and the shift from static to dynamic data [379].

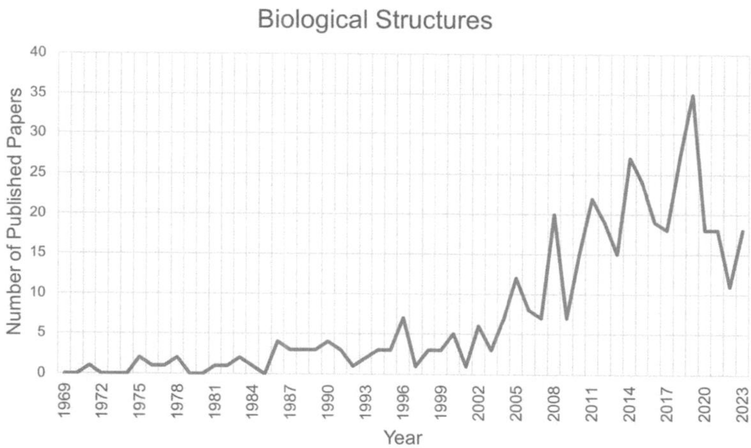

Fig. 3.10 Number of *biological structure visualization* papers published over time

3.4.1 Biomolecules: From Static to Dynamic Representations

The earliest systems focused on representing molecular structures using line-based, so-called *licorice* or *stick*, representations of atomic bonds [165, 597]. Within a decade, numerous systems appeared that complemented the stick models with *ball-and-stick* models, which included representations of atoms [272] and purely atomic models, which served as a simple space-filling representation of molecular volumes [588]. *CPK models* (named after chemists Corey, Pauling, and Koltun), which use van der Waals radii to represent atoms as spheres, have been employed. This representation is also referred to as *van der Waals surface*. Its simplicity makes it one of the most used molecular-surface representations to this day. Definitions that represent the molecules as smooth surfaces or better capture their physico-chemical properties were also introduced. This started with solvent accessible surfaces by

LEE and RICHARDS [360], and was followed by solvent excluded surfaces [115, 510], skin surfaces [148], and ligand excluded surfaces [378]. In addition to atomic and surface models, schematic representations of biomolecular entities and their secondary structures, called *cartoon* or *ribbon diagrams*, were proposed [511].

The earliest molecular visualizations used vector-based line graphics. They often employed illustrative techniques such as hatching to convey the 3D shape of a surface [398]. With advances in computer graphics hardware, raster-based algorithms appeared, and the research effort during the 1980s and 1990s was dedicated to improving the visual quality. Examples include lighting and shading, and speeding up of the rendering to achieve interactivity [542, 638]. Interactive molecular graphics strongly increased in popularity with GPU-based rendering starting in the early 2000s. At this time, the focus of research shifted from static data to dynamic representations. The molecular motion has been determined from molecular dynamics (MD) simulations. This further increased the need to improve rendering speed and over the past two decades, many approaches for rendering molecular structures were presented [79, 227, 324, 379]. Several works also focused on improving the *perceptual quality* of the results with techniques such as ambient occlusion [228, 582] (see Fig. 3.11), illumination models [230], depth of field effects [317], or transparency [229, 281]. Mapping of biochemical properties onto molecular representations was also studied. Cipriano and Gleicher [109] investigated a surface simplification in combination with glyphs for this purpose.

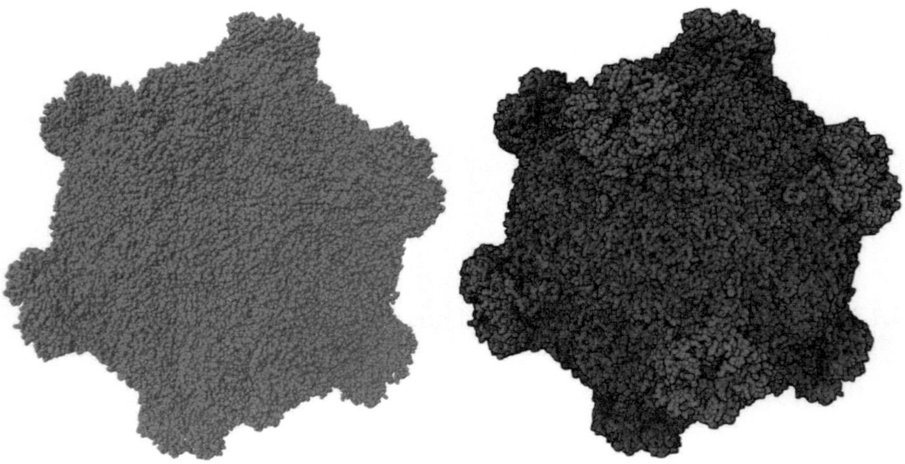

(a) (b)

Fig. 3.11 Visualization of the deformed wing virus (PDB ID: 5MV5) with basic shading (a) and with ambient occlusion and outlines, highlighting the virus structure (b). *Image created with Mol* Viewer* [562]

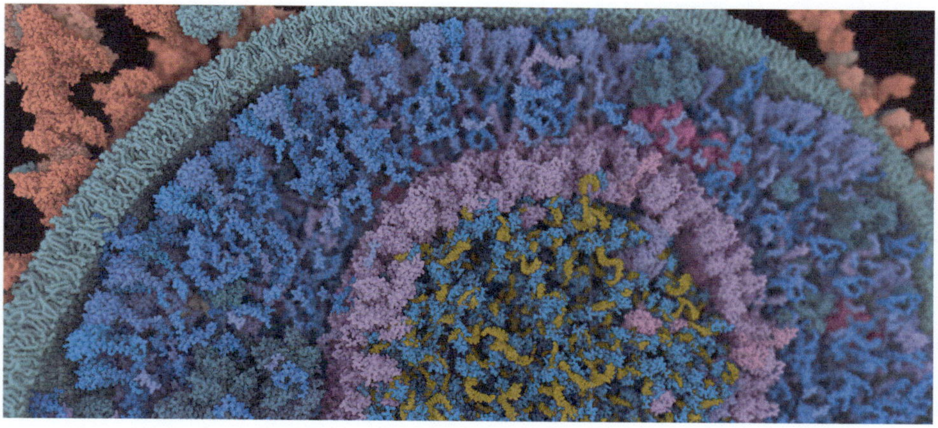

Fig. 3.12 Visualization of an HIV virion (*©2017 IEEE, Reprinted with permission from* [303])

In order to support better analysis of molecular motion, several methods for the explicit visualization of molecular flexibility have been developed. Backbone-thickness modulation and coloring are supported by multiple tools [130, 316]. Alternatively, arrow glyphs depict the direction and amount of motion [87]. Visual analytics tools for an in-depth analysis of molecular motion patterns were also presented [41].

In the last decade, we see another shift in data complexity, moving from the visualization of a single structure or small structure complexes towards the visualization of crowded biological environments (Fig. 3.12) [156, 273, 303, 358]. This brings further challenges, calling for level-of-detail strategies and multiscale approaches [211, 359]. To support scientific dissemination and education, storytelling and narrative approaches are being examined [318].

3.4.2 Analysis of Molecular Interactions

Advances in computational biology have also led to the development of specialized techniques and tools for drug design, protein engineering, and structural biology. Here the interactions of macromolecules play an important role, either with other macromolecules or with smaller molecules called ligands. *Molecular docking*, i.e., studying how molecular structures fit together, has thus been a prominent topic in molecular visualization.

Initial research of molecular interactions focused on 3D spatial representations of potential reaction sites [32, 361, 637], or the shape of transportation paths through the molecules [111, 326, 579] discussed in detail in the survey by Krone et al. [325]. Purely spatial representations were impractical for complex MD simulations. Thus, abstracted 2D representations [347, 640] and visual analytics systems were proposed. These typically combine spatial and abstract elements of important features, such as the width of a transportation path or binding energy. The goal is to navigate the domain scientists to interesting portions of the data. Systems investigating dynamic changes and properties of a single molecule [91, 377] were followed by tools for the analysis of MD simulations. These involve multiple entities [583], systems for examining protein-ligand docking simulations [146, 170, 460], flow of water molecules [631], or analysis of protein-lipid interactions [17].

3.4.3 Comparative and Abstracted Visualizations

Comparison of biomolecules is a common task in biochemistry research. It typically involves abstracted representations. One of the most common approaches is the comparison of aligned 1D sequences. Here, color is typically used to make the comparison easier. A 1D sequential representation is often used for mapping additional properties. In Aquaria [449] it is used for comparing protein secondary structures. Nowadays, similar representations can be found in protein databases, such as PDBsum [346]. Kocincová et al. [310] extended these methods by integrating information about the orientation of the secondary structures into the 1D representation. 2D schematic diagrams of molecular structures are frequently used in comparisons. For example, in LigPlot+ [347] they are utilized for the comparison of protein-ligand bindings. Other approaches in comparative visualization unfold or flatten molecular surfaces or parts thereof, such as binding sites [545] and transportation tunnels [314]. Schatz et al. [544] mapped the intricate molecular shape to a surrounding sphere, which was then unfolded using traditional cartographic map projections. For comparison and analysis of high-dimensional and ensemble data, such as drug discovery screening (Fig. 3.13), dimensionality reduction-based [535] and aggregation-based [168, 224] techniques were designed.

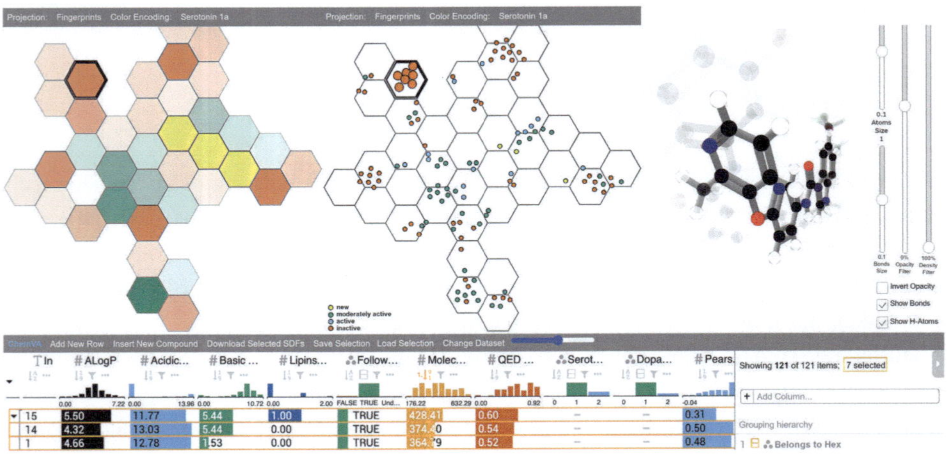

Fig. 3.13 Interface of ChemVA for analysis of chemical compounds in virtual screening. The hexagonal view showing compound distribution is complemented by a 3D view of selected compounds and a detailed table view (*©2020 IEEE, Reprinted with permission from:* [535])

3.4.4 Mixed Reality

The majority of visualization systems in biology and biochemistry is intended for desktop computers and standard I/O devices. However, already in the late 1990s, first virtual environments in biochemistry were introduced. The evolution followed the general progress of the technology, from stereoscopic displays [205] and CAVE environments [9], through haptic feedback devices [72, 219], to modern VR glasses [274]. Recurring topics included structural assembly [189], molecular docking [364], and interaction with MD simulations [319]. They all benefit from enhanced spatial perception in virtual environments. Other topics concern general data exploration and presentation techniques for education, which will be discussed in Sect. 3.9. Currently, the development of VR/AR techniques for biology and biochemistry is an active area of research. While some tools, such as UnityMol [388], are well established, techniques targeting novel research areas, such as DNA nanotechnology [339], are emerging.

3.4.5 Visual Analytics for Microscopy Imaging

The majority of previously discussed methods operated with data coming from computational simulations and modeling, but advances in imaging technologies, e.g., cryo-EM [30], are revolutionizing the way biological structures are obtained. Multiple visualization approaches were developed for the analysis of microscopy images. Early methods focused on the detection and subsequent visualization of structures of interest, predominantly cells, their properties, and temporal evolution. For this, techniques such as kymographs [369] or space-time cubes [627] were employed. Cell-lineage diagrams depicting important events, such as mitosis, were used to represent the developmental history of the cell population [96], while dimensionality reduction and clustering were employed to identify similar structures [214] in image datasets. Furthermore, many of the more recent approaches are used in gene expression analysis, and we discussed them in Sect. 3.3. Another area, where microscopy images play a crucial role is digital pathology. This is discussed in Sect. 3.5.

> *The approaches in Sect. 3.4 deal with spatial data. Over the years, the focus has shifted from* ***static to temporal and dynamic data,*** *all of which are at* ***molecular or cellular scale.*** *Target users of the presented methods are typically* ***researchers.*** *Visualizations commonly address* ***communication*** *as well as* ***analysis and exploration tasks.***

3.5 Visualization for Tumor Diagnosis and Treatment

In this section, we discuss approaches supporting registration and segmentation, and solutions facilitating tumor localization by focusing on diagnostics, tumor treatment, and clinical research. We discuss traditional 2D/3D strategies and, subsequently, multimodal or time-varying visual analytics approaches, and cohort-based implementations. In Fig. 3.14, we see that the topic dates back to the 1990s (when, for instance, the seminal papers of Levoy et al. appeared [367]), with a high peak just before 2010 [450]. This trend increases even further, due to the advent of artificial intelligence-related work.

3.5.1 Approaches Supporting Registration and Segmentation

Within the field of registration, an important aspect is the analysis and validation of the accuracy of registration methods. Hamdan et al. [213] propose checkerboard visualizations to verify the alignment of the registration between MRI and CT images. Visualization of registration quality incorporating local image dissimilarity metrics was proposed by Schlachter et al. [550]. Finally, RegistrationShop by Smit et al. [585] supports rigid and non-rigid volume registration using 3D visualizations and intuitive interactive tools that manipulate the volumes providing real-time visual feedback.

For the support of (semi-)automatic segmentations, three main sub-topics have been investigated in the past: aiding the segmentation of regions of interest, enhancing segmentation outcomes by post-processing, and assessing the outcome of the segmentation. In the first category, Raidou et al. [503] employ a visual analytics approach to improve classifier design for brain lesion detection using features derived from diffusion imaging. Torsney-Weir et

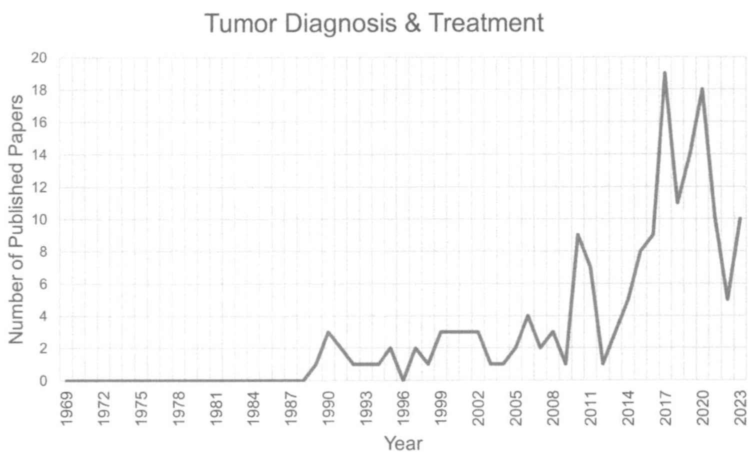

Fig. 3.14 Number of *tumor diagnosis and treatment* papers published over time

al. [624] propose a visual analysis tool to systematically explore the multi-dimensional parameter space impacting the quality of image segmentation algorithms. In the second category, Moench et al. [417, 421] present a modification to common mesh smoothing algorithms to preserve non-artifact features by focusing on previously identified staircase artifacts. In the third category, Reiter et al. [505] developed a web-based visual analytics approach to facilitate understanding how the shape and size of pelvic organs affect the accuracy of automatic segmentation methods. The approach also enabled quick identification of segmentation errors and their correlation to anatomical features.

3.5.2 Solutions Facilitating Tumor Localization

Diagnostics. Tumor diagnostics requires determining the location, extent (largest diameter or volume), subtype (tumor grading) of a tumor, and tumor staging. This process involves radiologic or nuclear image data, while tumor grading also requires microscopic data for characterizing tumor cells. To obtain an overview on the structure and location of tumors, volume rendering approaches were proposed [367, 551], also to support path planning [226].

Preim et al. [484] introduced resection proposals, i.e., visualizations of the resection area that is necessary for removing a tumor with a certain safety margin considering the vascular supply. Krüger et al. [329] investigated smart visibility techniques to reveal suspicious lesions for tumor surgery planning, particularly in the neck region. Preim et al. [492] developed measurement tools integrated into 3D visualizations to support tumor surgery planning. The extent of a tumor and distances to nearby structures at risk can be automatically presented.

Recent visualization and visual analytics approaches focus mainly on the analysis of the tumors prior to treatment or for supporting treatment decisions. In the former category, a special case is the work of Heckel et al. [222] where a sketch-based approach for the modification of tumor segmentations is proposed. There is also significant work with regard to tumor staging by Rössling et al. [528] and Pankau et al. [462]. Müller et al. [429] provide clinical decision-making support for tumor boards in a visual analytics design. It gives a visual summary of all evidence items and their relevance for the computation result, along with necessary textual information, for guided tumor staging.

Colonoscopy. In virtual colonoscopy, early approaches revolved around volume visualizations [246, 654, 681], especially in combination with extracting features, such as the lumen or the centerline of the colon, for polyp detection [100, 653]. Non-linear colon unfolding provided a better, more comprehensive view of the complex surface of the organ and on potential polyps [209, 645] (Fig. 3.15).

Real-time volume rendering for the generation of high-quality images of large volumetric colon data appeared in the early 2000s [370]. It evolved into a complete pipeline for virtual colonoscopy [248, 263] and supported later also the reconstruction of surfaces from acquired endoscopic videos [291]. This flow of work was driven by KAUFMANN and colleagues, opening up new possibilities in clinical diagnostics and generating significant

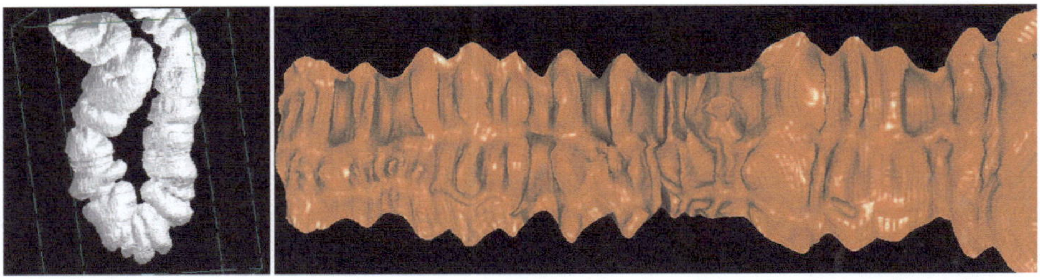

Fig. 3.15 3D view of the colon and virtual unfolding of a segment (*©2004 IEEE, Reprinted with permission from:* [645])

clinical contributions. Zhao et al. [688] proposed to automatically detect polyps using aggregates of surface shape information. The use of transfer functions for virtual colon cleansing was also investigated in real-time applications [533]. The capabilities of multiresolution GPU raycasting have been employed for real-time transfer function manipulation and fast multiresolution rendering. Recently, a volumetric-based VR immersive analytics application provided a wider field of view and field of regard for polyp search and analysis [413].

Pathology. In pathology, an early work by Leith et al. [362] focuses on cellular reconstruction, e.g., of astrocytes or tumor cells, for the communication of shape and substructure. The system supports contouring and visual representations, e.g., through surface rendering. In medical image analysis, pathology-related tasks, such as cell segmentation and analysis of histopathology images, were always a core topic. This has not been the case in the visualization domain. Recently, four main trends have been observed. First, we witness frameworks that deal with the interactive examination of large histopathology data either in the form of 2D image stacks [265] or in 3D, also in their native resolution [157]. Moreover, visual analytics approaches supporting pathologists with their diagnoses [119, 121, 122], also by linking to Electronic Health Records (EHRs) and biopsy data, have appeared. These may be extended to entire cohorts of patients [118, 120]. Furthermore, visual analytics approaches dealing with cellular and nuclear shape analysis [12] or with cellular screening and phenotype analysis [139, 327] are available. Visual analytics approaches that address spatially resolved omics data, bridging histopathology to other omics domains [590] have also been proposed. The latter two trends are the most recent ones, with works produced to date.

> *All approaches in Sect.* 3.5.2 *address* ***spatial data,*** *some of which are temporal or dynamic, and are* ***growing in dimensionality*** *over the years. The approaches deal with the* ***cellular or organism scale****. Most of the approaches target* ***researchers or practitioners*** *that are mainly interested in* ***analyzing*** *their own data.*

3.5.3 Strategies Aiding Tumor Treatment and Clinical Research

Tumor treatment involves a complex decision-making process. Treatment methods include surgery, radiation treatment, chemotherapy, tumor ablation, or immunotherapy. For each of these methods, many details need to be clarified prior to treatment. As an example, surgery may be more or less radical, and different access strategies need to be considered, affecting the risk of surgery and the risk of a recurrent tumor. On the other side, radiation treatment may be fractionated in a rather larger number of irradiation sessions, for which pre-operative planning is required [551].

Traditional 2D and 3D Approaches. Tumor treatment, and in particular radiation therapy, has vastly benefited from visual computing methods. In the 1980s, most of the approaches used in clinical practice to convey radiation information with respect to the patient's anatomy were limited to 2D slice-based views with additional contours for the organs and the dose fields. Significant contributions were made by LEVOY and INTERRANTE. Levoy et al. [367] proposed the first approach for 3D visualization targeting radiation therapy. A combination of surface and volume rendering was used to convey anatomy, treatment beams, and dose. Additionally, artistic stylizations were investigated to improve the perception of spatial relationships. A significant contribution is the introduction of the so-called "Beam's-eye view", which is used today in clinical practice. A few years later, Interrante and her colleagues investigated other volume rendering approaches for radiation treatment planning. They employed ridge-and-valley lines [255], curvature-directed strokes [256], and textures [257]. Although AR and VR methodologies have been applied to the domain of radiation therapy, they have not seen actual clinical adoption. An exception is VERT [659], a VR system targeting medical training.

Visual Analytics in Tumor Research. Challenging visualization problems in radiation therapy mainly concern supporting multimodal treatment planning [355, 549, 550], facilitating dose plan evaluation [163, 180], and enabling tumor characterization for personalized treatment. The most interesting evolution occurred in the latter direction—as approaches were mainly developed with exploratory and analytical tasks in mind to support the workflow of researchers. Early works focused on the segmentation and visualization of features derived from MRI perfusion data and were proposed by Coto et al. [123] (Fig. 3.16) and Oeltze et al. [450]. In the latter work, a visual analysis tool is presented that enables the exploration of correlations and relations between several features and parameters of perfusion data by using Principal Component Analysis (PCA) and multiple linked views. A survey on the visualization of perfusion data was authored by Preim et al. [487].

Subsequently, Fang et al. [159] built upon the concept of time activity curves. They propose methods to analyze and visualize time-varying multimodal data with adequate transfer functions. Intra-tumor classification has been discussed by Glasser et al. [196] for the division of a tumor into regions with distinct perfusion characteristics. Region merging is employed, which is summarized in a glyph-based representation for a fast overview of

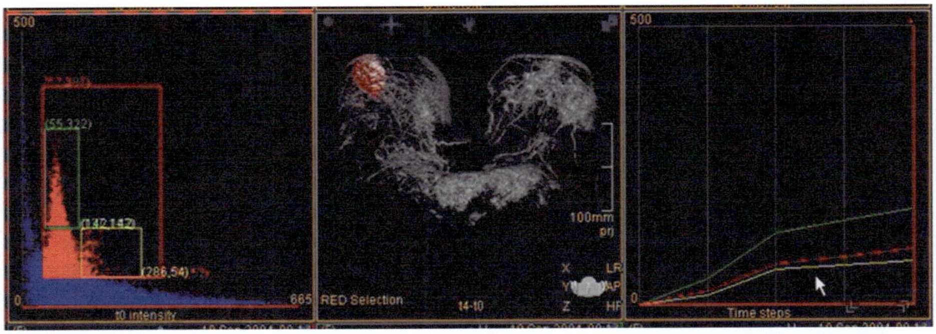

Fig. 3.16 The interactive visual system by Coto et al. [123] for the analysis of breast tumors using DCE-MRI data. *Original image created by Ernesto Coto*

an entire breast tumor. Nunes et al. [445] describe an integrated visual analytics framework enabling the multimodal fusion of MRSI data with PET and MRI data to gain insight into patient-specific tumor heterogeneity. Raidou et al. [502] enabled the identification of intra-tumor regions and the exploration of large multi-parametric cancer imaging data in comparison to clinical reference data. Recently, approaches address the integration of a large number of image-derived features for tumor characterization, such as the work of Mörth et al. [425, 426].

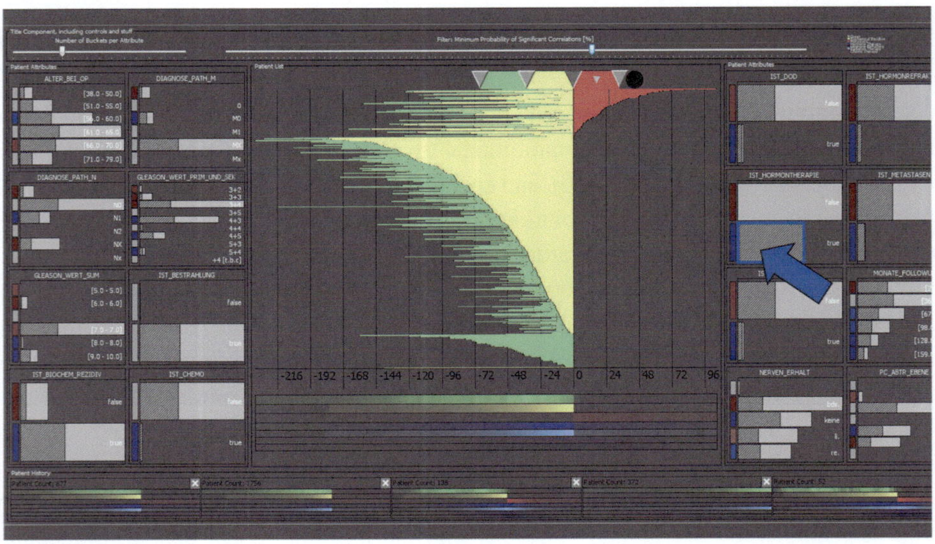

Fig. 3.17 The interactive visual system by Bernard et al. [49] enables to analyze cohorts of prostate cancer patients. *Image courtesy of Jürgen Bernhard, University of Zürich*

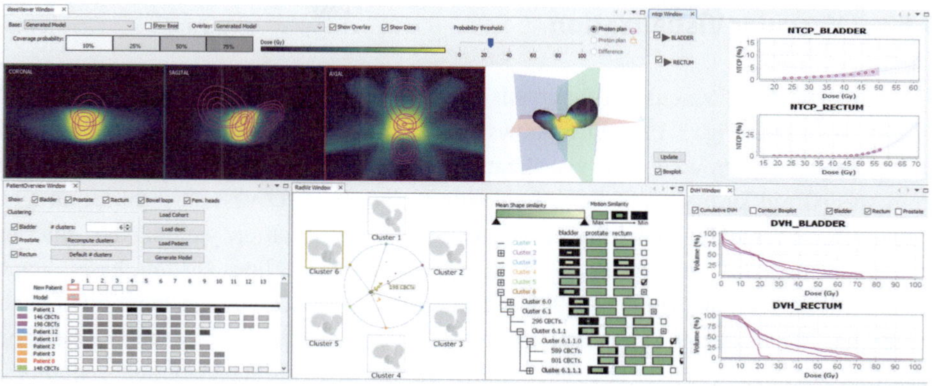

Fig. 3.18 PREVIS [169] employs changes during treatment from a retrospective cohort to build a generative model. It predicts how an incoming patient's anatomy will evolve during treatment. The model is interactively linked to treatment plan evaluation and supports domain experts in decision-making. *Image created by Katarína Furmanová, Masaryk University, for this book*

Cohort-based Approaches. A recent trend supports researchers to adapt radiotherapy through cohort-based visual analytics. An example is a system by Bernard et al. [49] for the visual analysis of high-dimensional patient attributes from a prostate cohort comprising many patient histories (Fig. 3.17). Other visual analytics tools account for anatomical variability to predict and prevent harm to the organs at risk close to the tumor. They range from single organ [500] to multi-organ approaches [167, 169] (Fig. 3.18). A recent cohort-based investigation by Wentzel et al. [666] proposes a visual computing approach for predicting treatment outcomes based on previously treated patient cohorts. Subsequently, Floricel et al. [162] proposed THALIS, a visual analytics approach targeting longitudinal-symptoms analysis in cancer therapy for new patients based on cases with similar diagnostic features and symptom evolution. We see a clear pattern going towards more complex data and tasks, i.e., going from the presentation of single-modality data, to multimodal or time-varying data exploration, and finally to the analysis of entire cohorts of patients to support research. A survey on visual computing methods in radiotherapy was provided by Schlachter et al. [551].

All approaches in Sect. 3.5.3 address ***spatial data,*** *some of which are* ***temporal or dynamic,*** *and are* ***growing in dimensionality*** *over the years. The approaches deal with the* ***organism scale,*** *and very recently moved on to* ***cohorts.*** *Most of the approaches target* ***researchers or practitioners*** *that conduct* ***exploratory, analytical, decision-making, and presentation tasks*** *with regard to their data.*

3.6 Vascular Visualization

The visualization of vascular structures is a classical medical visualization topic. This is evident also from Fig. 3.19, which shows the topic appeared already in the early 1990s and keeps steadily growing. The visualization of branching and elongated vessels benefits from specialized surface or volume rendering techniques. 3D vessel visualization techniques rely on vessel segmentation and often also on skeletonization, yielding the centerline and the local radius information for each point of the centerline. On this basis, graphics primitives, such as cylinders [397] and truncated cones [207], have been fitted to the centerline. The visualization based on truncated cones is an efficient trade-off between conflicting requirements, such as fast generation of the vascular tree, accuracy, and smoothness. It is available in MeVisLab and was the basis for a number of refinements, such as the illustrative techniques described in Sect. 3.6.2. Early techniques were not adapted to specific vessels and focused on surface rendering. An early survey article summarizes these developments [90].

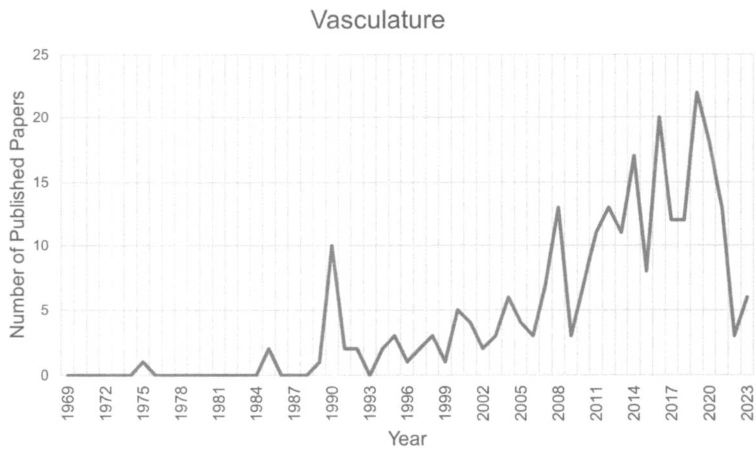

Fig. 3.19 Number of *vascular visualization* papers published over time

3.6.1 Explicit and Implicit Techniques

Explicit vessel visualization techniques are based on an explicit representation of the vessel geometry, e.g., through a polygonal surface mesh. Later these approaches were often replaced by *implicit* visualization techniques that enable a higher degree of smoothness. Examples for this category are *convolution surfaces* [451] and Multi-level Partition of Unity (MPU) Implicits [559]. Convolution surfaces were initially described by Bloomenthal as an implicit method to display skeletal primitives [60]. Thus, the method is applicable to the vessel centerline. Oeltze and Preim [451] adapted the method by using hierarchical data structures and techniques to further restrict the computation of the implicit function to narrow bands around the centerline. This was essential to apply the method to large vascular trees derived from CT and MRI data. Moreover, they adapted the reconstruction filter to achieve a correct representation of the local vessel diameter and to reduce the known "unwanted" effects of implicit surfaces.

Also, MPU implicits were not invented for displaying vascular structures, but to render large point sets resulting from scanning 3D geometries [453]. For vessel visualization, MPU implicits employ a point set derived by the vessel segmentation and provide piecewise quadratic approximations of the surface. They are more accurate compared to convolution surfaces and can represent also arbitrary cross-sections. Convolution surfaces assume circular cross-sections and thus cannot display pathologies. This line of research continued, e.g., with adaptive meshing strategies that consider curvature and view directions [678] and *sweep surfaces* as a strategy to generate watertight meshes [322]. Another essential development was presented by Mistelbauer et al. [415]. They approximate branches of vasculature by elliptical Fourier descriptors. These are more accurate than the circular cross-section assumption of convolution surfaces and enable smoother visualizations than methods without any model assumption. Implicit techniques tend to be computationally more intense than explicit approaches despite acceleration strategies. Bounding volumes and hierarchical data structures restrict the computation of the implicit function to narrow regions around the vessels.

3.6.2 Illustrative Techniques

Starting with the pioneering work from RITTER and HANSEN [216, 519] at Fraunhofer MEVIS, illustrative techniques were combined with vessel visualization to improve shape and depth perception. *Depth-encoding hatching* [519] and *supporting lines* connecting landmarks on a vessel tree with their shadow projection [352] are examples for this line of research. In the same vein, special color scales, such as pseudo-chromadepth, were developed to map depth onto a vascular tree and enhance its depth perception [527] (Fig. 3.20). The effectiveness of such techniques was assessed with depth judgment tasks. The focus was the *perceptual quality* of the visualizations.

3.6.3 Volume Rendering

The techniques described in Sects. 3.6.1 and 3.6.2 require a vessel segmentation and often lose smaller branches of vascular trees as they are very difficult to segment. It is promising to employ direct volume rendering based on the original data. This requires also some

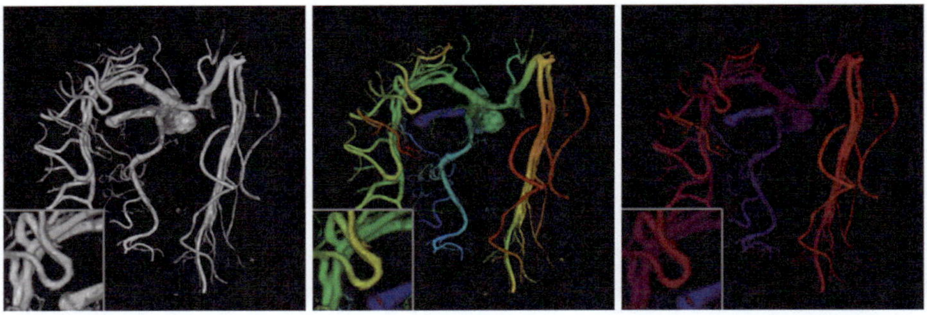

(a) regular coloring (b) chromadepth (c) pseudo chromadepth

Fig. 3.20 Depth cues through color coding. The depth is not encoded in the color (a), chromadepth (b), pseudo-chromadepth reduced to red and blue (c). (*©2006 Springer Nature, Reprinted with permission from* [527] *and* Springer Nature)

preprocessing, such as *vesselness filtering*, and the adjustment of appropriate transfer functions. An essential work in this area was carried out by Joshi et al. [278] who also employed adapted color scales to support depth perception. Even earlier, 2D transfer functions (using intensity and gradient magnitude) were designed for enhancing vascular structures [233]. An essential article about transfer functions for vessel visualizations with a sound theoretical basis was provided by Laethen et al. [348]. A summary of vessel visualization with volume rendering is provided by Kubisch et al. [331].

3.6.4 Projection-Based Methods

Most of the techniques described so far aim at surgery planning, giving an overview of vascular trees, and a clear depiction of branchings, e.g., close to a tumor that should be removed. For the diagnosis of vascular diseases, projection-based methods are more appropriate. They are often referred to as *vessel maps*, employing the metaphor of a (cartographic) map.

An essential technique is *curved planar reformations* (CPRs) that summarize the whole course of a vessel, e.g., in the legs. This technique was introduced by Achenbach et al. [2] and later refined by Kanitsar, Fleischmann and colleagues [287, 288] (Fig. 3.21). They introduced CPR variants that summarize whole vascular trees instead of just one vessel segment [524]. The development of CPRs is a true success story since these techniques are now widely used in clinical practice and radiology textbooks explain how to interpret them. One problem that remains with conventional CPR is the need to rotate around the centerline of a vessel. Mistelbauer et al. [414] introduced Curvicircular Feature Aggregation where the rotated images are summarized in a single view. This enables a faster diagnosis, however, the resulting single-image visualization can easily get quite complex.

Many more recent map-based vessel visualizations were developed, including those that present the vascular anatomy along with scalar attributes, such as wall thickness or simulated pressure on the wall. Some map-based techniques even convey the internal blood flow [43]. Such visualizations are referred to as *flow maps*. EULZER and colleagues recently provided a survey on *vessel maps* [153].

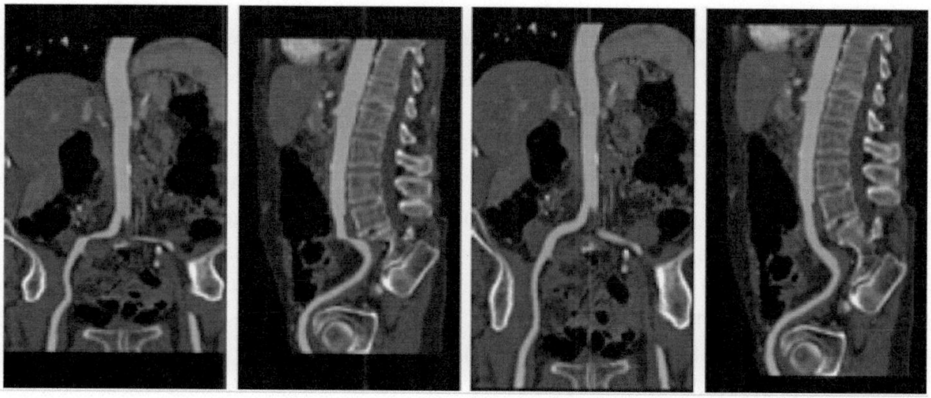

(a) (b) (c) (d)

Fig. 3.21 Curved planar reformations [286]: (a), (b) Projected, (c), (d) Stretched. *Image distributed under the terms of the* Creative Commons CC BY 4.0 *license*

3.6.5 Specialized Vessel Visualization

Most research on the visualization of vessel structures was independent of a specific diagnostic or treatment planning task. However, some authors developed visualization techniques specifically intended for cerebral vascular structures. Hastreiter et al. [220] pioneered volume rendering of vascular structures. They designed transfer functions for emphasizing aneurysms and focusing on their local environment. Puig et al. [496] developed a comprehensive system for visualizing the cerebral arteries with surface-based methods after vessel segmentation. Later, Miao et al. [411] designed an abstract representation for visual quantification of cerebral arteries. Specific solutions were also developed for the diagnosis of coronary heart disease (CHD). Termeer et al. [616] presented a volumetric extension of the bull's eye plot to incorporate additional information into the plot. The solution developed by Glaßer et al. [195] for CHD employs the result of a previous segmentation. Based on histogram analysis of the involved voxels, a transfer function simultaneously shows the vessel surface and inner structures, such as stents or plaques.

3.6.6 Visualization of Vasculature and Embedded Flow

For the diagnosis of vascular diseases, e.g., for the assessment of severity and associated risk, there is an increasing interest in blood flow. Blood flow may be simulated with computational fluid dynamics (CFD). These simulations tend to increase in precision these days since the underlying simulation models are more refined than in the past. Blood flow in large vessels, in particular in the aorta, can also be measured with 4D PC-MRI, a variant of MR imaging. Blood flow needs to be visualized along with the surrounding vascular surfaces. Several attempts were made to design visualizations that faithfully convey both the vascular surface and the internal flow.

Using vascular surface models for CFD simulations requires smooth geometric models and a high triangle quality, i.e., almost equilateral triangles. Moreover, the size of the triangles should not change abruptly. Artifacts from medical imaging, such as beam hardening, also need to be corrected to ensure that the iterative solution of the underlying equation system converges and to avoid misleading simulation results. A key role in the process of preparing vascular surface models for simulation plays the Vascular Modeling Toolkit (VMTK) [21] that is publicly available and frequently employed.

Gasteiger et al. [178] developed a technique based on Fresnel shading where the vessel wall is enhanced, whereas regions of the vessel surface that would occlude the internal flow are rendered with increased transparency. Lawonn et al. [349] refined this method and enable also the display of time-dependent flow (Fig. 3.22). Later, they refined these methods further by depicting also the locally varying wall thickness as another essential parameter to assess the rupture risk of an aneurysm [350] (Fig. 3.23).

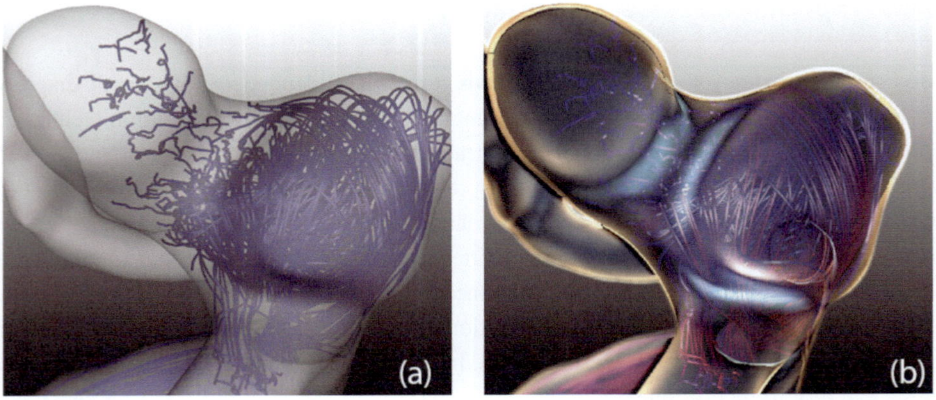

Fig. 3.22 Integral curve displays are frequently embedded in a semi-transparent rendering of the vessel wall (a). Improved perception of surface depth and shape while maintaining flow visibility is achieved based on a view-dependent emphasis of feature lines (b) *(From:* [349], *©John Wiley & Sons Inc., 2014)*

3.6.7 Mapping Features on Vascular Surfaces

For advanced diagnosis and medical research, it may be beneficial to display vascular structures along with features that characterize locally changing values, such as the thickness of the vessel wall. Features can also be derived from a blood flow simulation, e.g., the wall shear stress (WSS) that indicates the pressure on the vessel wall. This parameter is associated with the rupture risk. Features may be mapped to color or to textures. To display several parameters at once, e.g., wall thickness and wall shear stress, is particularly challenging. Neugebauer et al. [431] designed a map-based visual representation that gives an overview on an entire aneurysm with its inflow and outflow region and maps WSS to colors. Behrendt et al. [42] presented a 3D visualization of the cerebral arteries such that color can be used to support depth perception and a feature can be overlaid onto the vessel surface.

3.6.8 Visualization and Exploration of Blood Flow

Starting around 2008, several groups made contributions to an efficient exploration of simulated or measured blood flow [617]. Advanced blood flow visualizations include a number of illustrative techniques [69, 635]. Exploration involves appropriate interaction techniques to restrict the flow to interesting parts or to focus the flow visualization. Examples include: probing the flow with an appropriate widget [636], the use of line predicates [68], lens-based interaction [177], and transfer function-based techniques to emphasize, e.g., slow or fast flow [432]. Moreover, special methods to emphasize near-wall flow were developed since such flow interacts with the vessel wall directly and thus is particularly interesting [433].

Some authors also applied feature detection and classification methods to focus the visualization of blood flow on these features. This is also motivated by a large number of medical publications that classify flow (manually) based on the occurrence and type of vortices, e.g., correlating the size of vortices, their location, and orientation (clockwise or counterclockwise) with the presence of a disease. Köhler et al. [312] integrated vortex detection methods in the visualization of blood flow and Meuschke et al. [404] classified vortices according to medical publications, e.g., into clockwise or counterclockwise flow (Fig. 3.24).

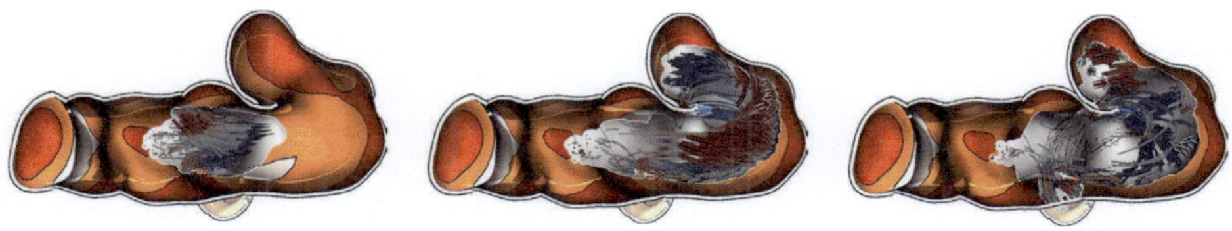

Fig. 3.23 A GPU-based implementation of a visualization proposed by Lawonn et al. facilitates wall thickness analysis through real-time rendering and flexible interactive data exploration mechanisms (*©2015 IEEE, Reprinted with permission from:* [350])

The semi-automatic classification could be a considerable improvement over the subjective manual classification.

3.6.9 From Individuals to Populations

The most recent trend in the visualization of vascular structures and blood flow is to consider whole groups of patients, healthy volunteers, or even the comparison between whole groups. A clinical motivation is to characterize similarities and differences, e.g., between aging persons and patients with a certain disease or gender-specific differences. In particular, for blood flow-related measurements and features, the ranges of *normal* values are still not clear, which is also a consequence of non-standardized image acquisition procedures. Meuschke et al. [403] introduced a system for exploring a database of patients with cerebral aneurysms and the associated blood flow. Automatically defined previews for each patient support patients selection and a number of views enable their comparison. The GUCCI (Guided Cardiac Cohort Investigation)-framework [405] serves to analyze and compare groups of patients together with their aortic blood flow. As an example, the flow is investigated at six standardized planes located at anatomical landmarks, as they are widely used in medical research. The major results are summarized in a glyph-based visualization, which enables to present the results for a moderate number of patients.

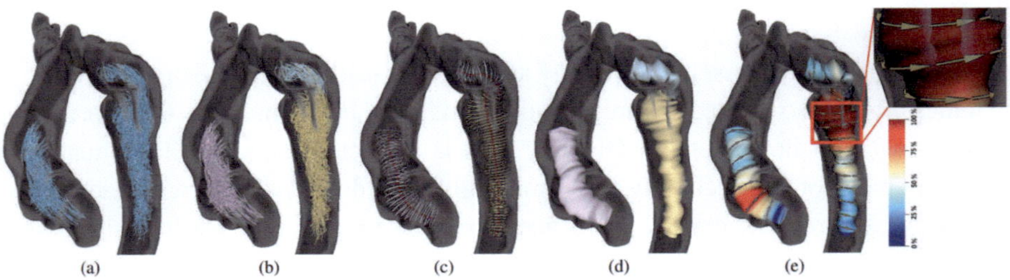

Fig. 3.24 3D glyph-based vortex visualization. The vortex-representing path lines (a) are clustered (b). For each cluster, a cubic spline (red) is calculated, and at each spline point an ellipse approximates the local vortex expansion (c). The ellipses are triangulated to a surface (d) on which the blood flow features are depicted using color coding and arrow glyphs (e) (*©2016 IEEE, Reprinted with permission from:* [404])

All approaches in Sect. 3.6 *address* ***spatial data,*** *which have* ***grown in dimensionality*** *over the years. The most recent approaches have moved to* ***vector-based*** *solutions and deal with* ***temporal or dynamic data****. The approaches deal with the*

organism**—and few, see Sect. 3.6.9, with the **cohort scale**. The users are **researchers or practitioners** that are mainly conducting **analytical or decision-making tasks.

3.7 Visualizing the Brain

In this section, we review the evolution of visualization approaches dedicated to brain anatomy, activity, and connectivity (at a macro- and micro-scale). Work on cerebrovascular visualization, and brain- or neurosurgery is discussed in Sects. 3.6 and 3.8, respectively. In Fig. 3.25, we see that the topic dates back to the late 1980s. There is a steep increase through the years starting in the 2000s—due to new acquisition modalities that allowed us to move from the visualization of the brain anatomy [573] to tensor [342] or multimodal data [374], and finally to investigate the brain at a microscopic scale [51, 84].

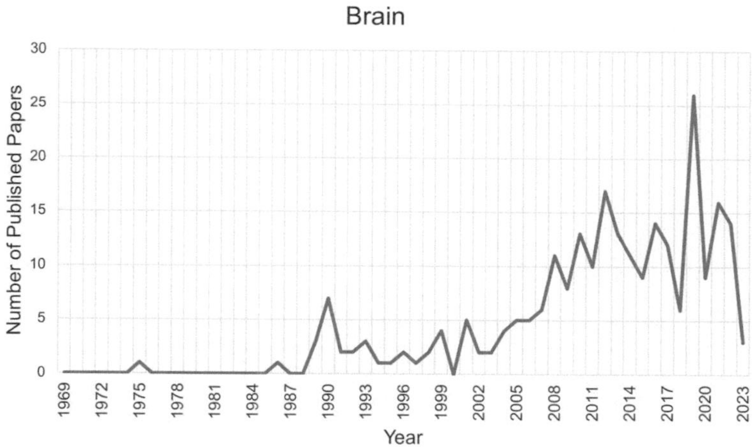

Fig. 3.25 Number of *brain visualization* papers published over time

3.7.1 Visualizing the Anatomy of the Brain

From Single-modality to Multi-modality Approaches. With papers as early as 1986 [560], visualizing the anatomy of the brain has been one of the first research directions pursued by our community. Early approaches focused more on investigating methods for the accurate extraction [466, 560] and expressive rendering of brain shapes [685]. They addressed the needs of researchers for the representation or communication of brain structures. This was later revisited in the context of multimodal [374, 602, 632] or multichannel MR [335] visualization, and also in combination with functional information. This concerns either activity information [203, 260] (Sect. 3.7.2) or connectivity information [50, 253] (Sect. 3.7.3).

From here on, approaches are moving towards helping researchers explore and analyze their data as well. Combining MRI and PET images for volume rendering was initially investigated in the 1990s [184, 633]. These early approaches focused on understanding the underlying anatomy and pathologies, such as tumors. Visualization was also used as a means to facilitate registration [184]. Multimodal visualization has also been investigated for the comparative assessment of multiple segmentations from brain data [374]. The linked analysis of brain imaging and clinical measurements of activity was recently re-investigated for supporting hypothesis generation and reasoning in cohort studies [276] (Fig. 3.26).

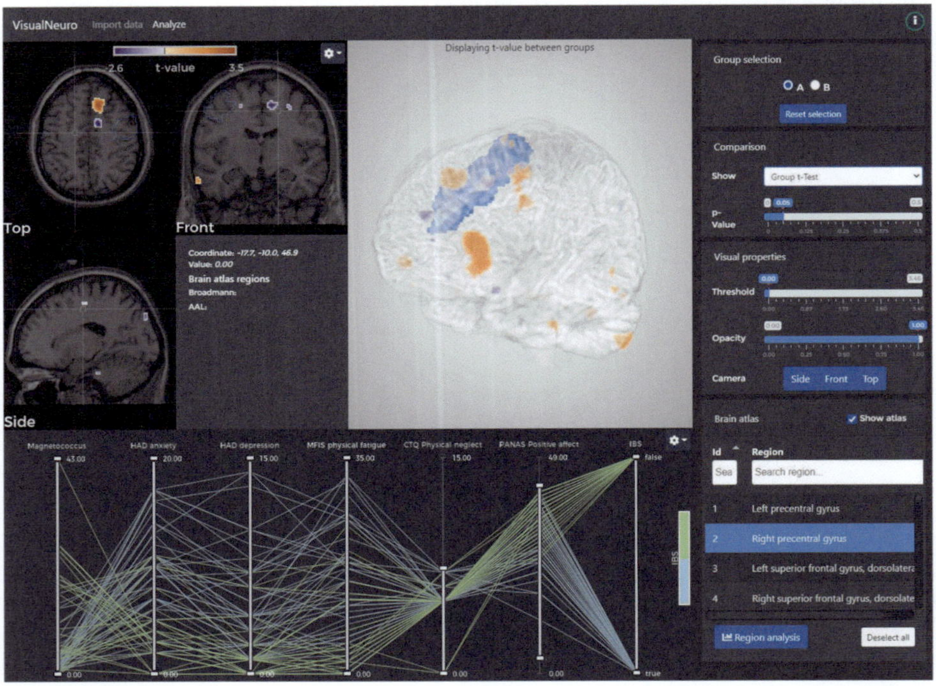

Fig. 3.26 Overview of a visual environment for the combined exploration of fMRI and multivariate clinical data proposed by Jönsson et al. [276]. Parallel coordinates support the selection of subject groups, while spatial views support the representation of differences. *Image courtesy of Daniel Jönsson, Linköping University*

Communicating Anatomy with Brain Atlases. Visualizing the anatomy of the brain resulted also in brain atlases for teaching, medical training, and scientific communication [97, 573]. In particular, the Harvard Brain Atlas [573] included automated segmentation methods, slice editing, interactive definition of neuroanatomical regions of interest, and 3D surface rendering techniques to provide a digital brain for teaching purposes. More recently, the feasibility of generating realistic models of anatomy based on cadaveric dissections has been investigated [97]. The added value of such models has been evaluated for anatomy education and training simulators. All these approaches target mainly scientific communication and training.

Reformation-based Approaches. In Sect. 3.6.4, we discussed projection-based methods for the visualization of vascular structures. Similar approaches have also been used to represent and visually simplify brain structures, and we often refer to them as *brain reformations* [20, 254]. An example is applications for the comparative assessment of inter-species brain structures [560, 594]. These early approaches focused on supporting the visual communication of structures to researchers or practitioners. This changed later to integrate more explorative or analytical environments. An example visualizes curvilinear reformatting for displaying the cerebral anatomy through a 3D painting metaphor [576]. The goal is to define the reference surface that the user sees, while an animation of the reformatting is generated at an interactive frame rate. For large-scale applications in neuroanatomy research, a framework for data processing, mining, and visualization of brain structures has been developed. It also allows for comparative analyses with respect to existing atlases [279]. Intuitive visualizations for high-level user queries further support an ontology-based exploration of hierarchical surface-based neuroanatomical atlases [338].

Most of the approaches in Sect. 3.7.1 deal with ***static and scalar spatial data*** *with only a few dynamic solutions (those that relate to VR/AR approaches). We mainly encounter* ***low-dimensional,*** *and only recently multi-dimensional data of the brain (****organism scale****). Most of the work targets* ***researchers*** *as users. Initially, the work was intended for* ***communication tasks,*** *then evolved to cover also* ***exploration and analysis.***

3.7.2 Visualizing the Activity of the Brain

Brain cells communicate through electrical activity, which can be recorded using electroencephalograms (EEG). An EEG uses electrodes to capture brainwave activity, and each electrode provides measurements for an EEG channel. Nowadays, EEGs can have as many as 256 channels. Tracking and displaying the electrical activity of the brain, in the form of wave patterns, was initially investigated in 1975 to quickly calculate parametrizations of the analysis [185]. Later, approaches focused also on practical use, providing support for diagnostic work that encapsulated both processing and display of the waves [114]. This was in addition to their usage in neurophysiological research. Afterward, visualization in phase space was also made possible [493]. Spatio-temporal dynamics in EEG data started to become an active field of research in the late 1980s [138].

Multi-channel data came into focus only in the late 2000s with multi-dimensional representations, such as parallel coordinates [614], and graph layouts [124, 615]. Ten Caat et al. [615] developed an approach that was 100,000 times faster than previously proposed methods for 128 channels. It also supports group analysis employing user-determined, hypothesis-driven regions of interest (ROIs), called Functional Units (FU). This was later extended with graph averaging [124] to provide comparative functionalities for determining which brain regions are more commonly involved in a certain task. To extract and visualize meaningful and common neural activity patterns across areas of the brain, Anderson et al. [124] presented an analysis system for neuroscientists.

More advanced approaches to process dynamic multichannel data and coherence networks [266, 267] were published only a few years ago. Remarkably a direction for future work as pointed out by ten Caat et al. [615] in 2008 concerning specific ROIs in brain maps, has finally been explored in 2020 by Bayrak et al. [38]. The method gives neuroscientists definition and analysis of functionalities by clustering temporally correlated brain parcellations, i.e., distinct brain partitions, from atlases.

The approaches in Sect. 3.7.2 deal with ***spatial and abstract data****—most of which are* ***dynamic and multi-dimensional data*** *of brain activity (****organism scale****). Most of the work targets* ***practitioners*** *as users, and recently there has been work also addressing* ***clinical research.*** *The work covers mostly* ***exploration and analysis tasks****, and only a few, older approaches are for communication purposes.*

3.7.3 Visualizing the Connectivity of the Brain

Macroscale Connectivity Visualization. Imaging and visualizing the macroscale connectivity of the brain is heavily based on the concept of capturing the free vs. obstructed diffusion of water molecules in tissues. In early visualization research, diffusion data has been reduced to scalar indices and treated as any other scalar-based dataset [302]. For example, Wenger et al. [665] used accelerated volume rendering through texture mapping to show fibers in the brain. Tensor glyphs appeared in 1996, when Pierpaoli et al. [476] proposed ellipsoid glyphs for representing diffusion anisotropy, which is a manifestation of tissues obstructing the otherwise free diffusion of water molecules. Soon after, Laidlaw et al. [342] developed smart normalization approaches to fit more glyphs into one view.

Weinstein et al. [663] explored the tracking, extraction, and visualization of tensor fields through tensor-lines, opening directions for the representation of tensor fields with streamtubes and streamsurfaces [687]. The two directions kept growing in parallel to each other. The work of KINDLMANN [301] is highly influential, where superquadrics are proposed as parameterized graphical objects to describe a single diffusion tensor. An example using superquadric glyphs (with different placements) is depicted in Fig. 3.27. Concerning fiber tracking, Vilanova et al. [643] investigated the seeding-based generation of streamlines to control clutter and reduce expensive computations. As an indication of the fast evolution, the aforementioned works, which are just a small subset of the literature, cover only a time span of eight years.

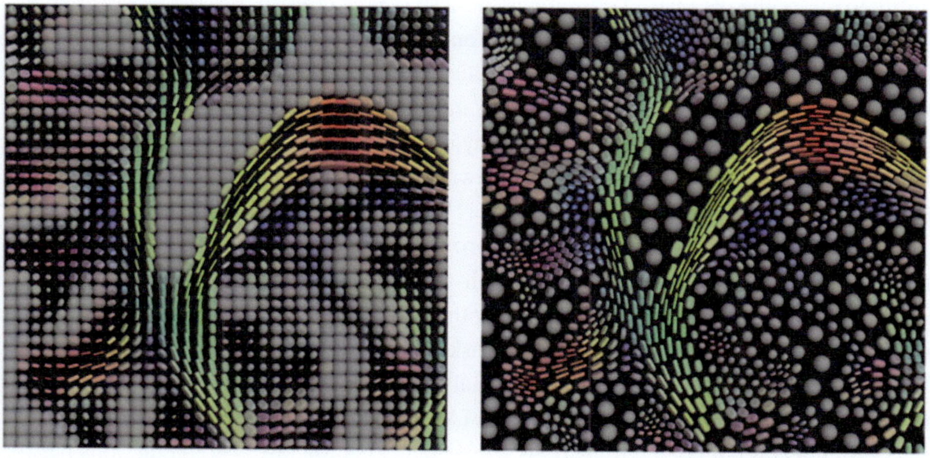

(a) Glyph placement on a regular grid (b) Glyph placement with packing

Fig. 3.27 Superquadric glyph placement (a) on a regular grid and (b) with packing. Glyph packing supports the visibility of anatomical structures better than a regular grid *(From:* [557], *©John Wiley & Sons Inc., 2018)*

The early approaches targeted the inspection of the macroscale connectivity of the brain, i.e., served mainly communication and presentation purposes. In the following years, both glyph-based and fiber-tracking techniques evolved to support accelerated computations and rendering. Glyphs have been used since then in comparative scenarios. Initially, this happened through juxtaposition [250, 556] and more recently through superimposition [1], and explicit encoding [684]—even for cohort studies [683]. To resolve visual clutter (and computation issues) due to the high density of fiber data, fiber tracking proposed solutions based on, e.g., bundling [75, 76], interaction [57], or 2D embeddings [268, 269]. Fiber tracking was also proposed to alleviate depth perception issues [458, 606] or deal with uncertainty [76, 556, 558]. These developments supported exploratory or analytical tasks, on top of presentation purposes. An overview of techniques for diffusion MRI visualization was authored by Schultz and Vilanova [557].

Microscale Connectivity Visualization. Imaging a cubic millimeter of brain tissue using serial Electron Microscopy (EM) produces data sets up to 800 TB of size [474], creating many computational challenges. Before 2000, connectomics analysis, i.e., extracting, visualizing, and analyzing connectivity of the brain at a micro-scale, focused on the segmentation of high-resolution EM data. The goal has been a quantitative analysis of segmented structures, such as measuring length, surface, or volume [194]. With the advancements in computational power and graphics, a whole range of new possibilities emerged to support neurobiology and neuroscience research. Bruckner's BrainGazer [84] first addressed the study of neural circuits through confocal microscopy and annotated anatomical structures, providing the ability to query the data based on semantic and spatial criteria.

Influential work by HADWIGER, BEYER, and PFISTER focused on exploring the general morphology of the data and on providing a scalable visualization of the original or segmented electron microscopy data [52, 206, 264]. For instance, ConnectomeExplorer [51] supported the exploration of high-resolution EM data by integrating a domain-specific query language into a scalable volume visualization framework. Simultaneously, visual metaphors such as circuit diagrams [592] or subway maps [10] that highlight synaptic connections were proposed. Sorger et al. [592] developed neuroMap to visualize nerve cell connectivities in the fruit fly brain as an interactive 2D graph. Neurolines [10] allows the user to view the connectivity between neurons by abstracting them to 2D straightened skeletons. Neurolines was the first system targeting comparative tasks.

More recently, approaches focus on the analysis of structures related to the brain's energy metabolism. For example, Mohammed et al. [419] explored 2D visual abstractions to allow for continuous user-specified transitions between abstraction levels in interactions between neurites and glial cells. Agus et al. [7] enable neuroscientists to investigate energy consumption in relation to brain morphology with a focus on glycogen granules.

Also, visual analytics tools have been developed in this area. An example is Facetto [327], which investigates hierarchical clustering of cell types for phenotype analysis. BrainTrawler [172] provides a web-based environment for the exploration of multiscale brain network data, while helping also the genetic analysis of brain networks. Recently, Barrio was proposed by Troidl et al. [626], as a scalable comparative approach (Fig. 3.28). It assists neuroscientists in the comparison of spatial neighborhoods by means of small multiples of spatial 3D views as well as abstract quantitative views. A recent survey on high-resolution brain connectomics has been written by Beyer et al. [55].

> *The approaches in Sect.* 3.7.3 *deal mostly with* ***multi- or high-dimensional spatial data*** *at an* ***organism scale.*** *Most of the work targets* ***researchers as users.*** *Initially, the work was intended for* ***communication tasks,*** *then evolved towards* ***exploration and analysis.***

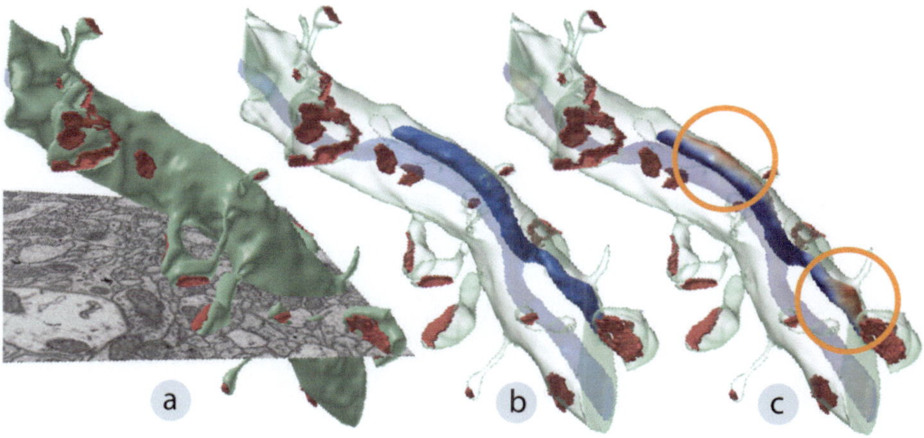

Fig. 3.28 Detailed 3D neighborhood view of BARRIO [626]. Depicted is a dendrite (green) and close synapses (red). (a) 2D slice overlay of the original EM data to show biological context. (b) Silhouette enhancing, and semi-transparent surface rendering to highlight how enclosed mitochondria (blue) are positioned within the dendrite. (c) Color-coding of a mitochondrion showing the distance between the mitochondrion and its surrounding cell membrane (*From:* [626], ©*John Wiley & Sons Inc., 2022*)

3.8 Visualization for Surgery

In this section, we discuss how visual computing and visualization approaches have supported the three main steps of a surgical procedure: pre-operative planning, intra-operative guidance, and post-operative assessment. This part includes a vast corpus of literature with a broad range of techniques. We do not differentiate based on the specific type of surgery, and the works discussed in the following may refer to approaches for neurosurgery, tumor ablations or removals, or endoscopic and laparoscopic procedures. In Fig. 3.29, we see that the topic dates back to the early 1980s through the 1990s [298], with a stable increase through the years—being a core topic of visualization.

3.8.1 Pre-operative Planning

Most surgical procedures require thorough pre-operative planning to ensure successful outcomes. Not surprisingly, surgical planning is one of the earliest and most researched topics for many domains of visual computing and visualization. KIKINIS, PREIM, and BARTZ were the first to investigate how visual computing could support surgical planning. Kikinis et al. [298] proposed an MRI-based atlas for surgical planning, model-driven segmentation, and teaching. Preim et al. [491] addressed planning of soft-tissue operations from the interaction point-of-view, as for example in oncologic liver and lung surgery.

In neurosurgery, multimodal volume visualizations facilitate the optimal therapeutic strategy by supporting the skull incision tailored to the underlying pathology, visualizing super-

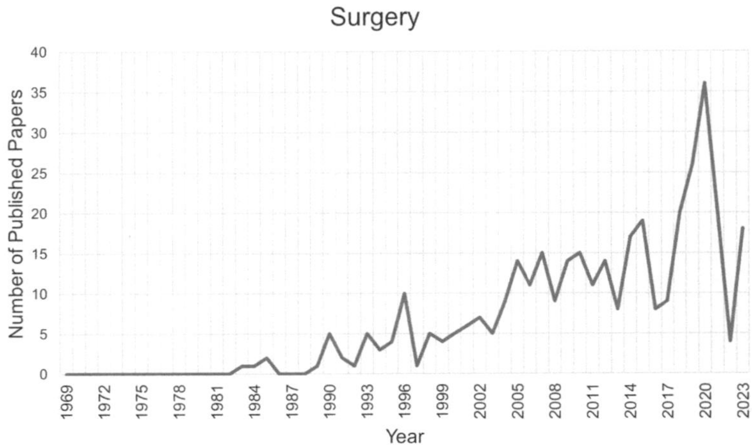

Fig. 3.29 Number of *surgery*-related papers published over time

ficial brain anatomy, and planning how to reach deep-brain lesions [54]. Subsequently, approaches were proposed that made use of expressive visualization at interactive frame rates [513]. This has been extended to generate fast volume renderings of anatomical structures with inhomogeneous pathological tissues by combining several MRI sequences [514]. Schulte zu Berge et al. [48] propose an approach for supporting navigation in multimodal neuro data sets during planning. This work comprises a force-directed graph model to overview the topology of the electrode map, integrates EEG, anatomical and functional data, and supports annotations through glyphs.

Uncertainty is important but is often avoided in pre-operative planning, as it is hard to quantify and introduces an additional level of complexity. One recent work [517] deals with uncertainty in ablation to show potential risks during the procedure. Real-time GPU implementations were proposed by Diepenbrock et al. [136] to convey the relation between lesions and various structures at risk, while also depicting potential uncertainty. Another work [135] is related to the 2010 SciVis Contest and suggests a workflow for the interactive support concerning brain tumor resection. The authors make use of a series of visualizations that allow experts to inspect the tumor and the access path. Krüger et al. [328] also discuss anatomical variability as uncertainty in the context of GPU volume rendering for endoscopic sinus surgery. GPU implementations have also been adopted for orthopedic surgery, where Dick et al. [134] propose an approach to support optimal implant design and position in hip-joint replacement planning that can immediately react to changes in the simulated stress tensor field.

A technique that bridges pre-operative planning with intra-operative guidance was proposed by Hansen et al. [215] for the simultaneous visualization of pre-operative planning models and intra-operative 2D ultrasound for open liver surgery. Illustrative approaches, as well as model-based risk analysis, have been later proposed for liver surgery [216, 217], while a training system was provided by Mönch et al. [420] (Fig. 3.30). Vascular analysis has also been considered [563]. Mühler and Preim [428] investigated the concept of reusable visualizations and animations to support surgical planning. The goal is to save time by generating the visuals once and reusing them for similar cases.

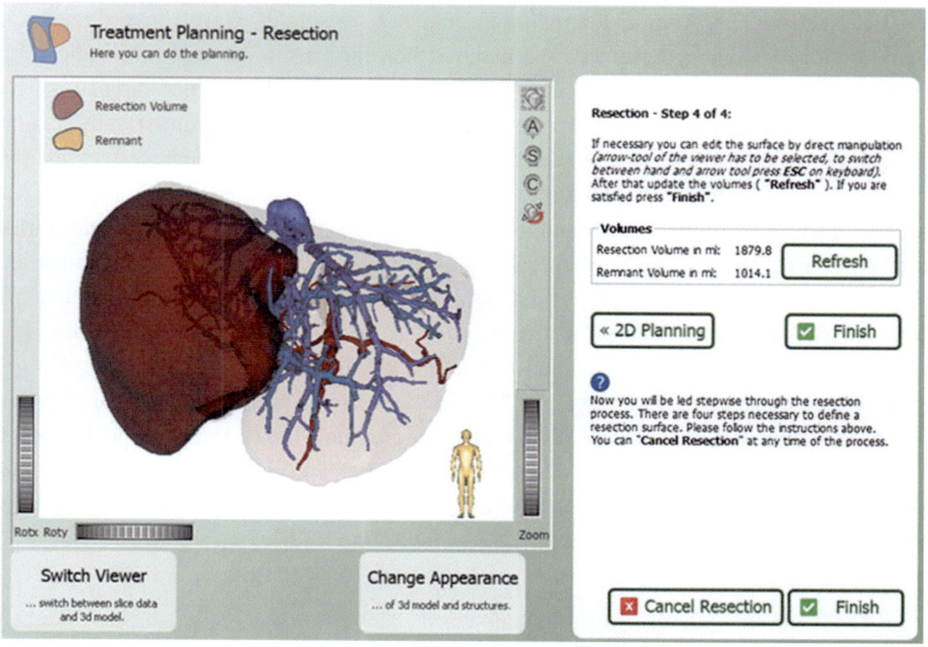

Fig. 3.30 THE LIVERSURGERYTRAINER: After the 2D planning, the result is presented in 3D for validation (resection volume: red, veins: blue, hepatic artery: red) with quantitative information on the right (*©2013 Springer Nature, Reprinted with permission from* [420] *and* Springer Nature)

Olofsson et al. [455] proposed a haptic interface for dose planning in stereo-tactic radiosurgery. Lundström et al. [387] introduced a multi-touch table for surgical planning and applied their system to orthopedic surgery. Another collaborative table-top display—but in VR—for neurosurgical planning was proposed by Eagleson et al. [147]. Recently, VR and AR have made a comeback also in surgery, with the latest works dealing with liver surgery in a collaborative planning environment in VR [106] or craniotomy in AR, making use of tracking accuracy information [673].

3.8.2 Intra-operative Guidance

In intra-operative guidance, NAVAB and HANSEN have had significant contributions. The majority of works on this topic are AR/VR approaches to guide interventions, multimodal approaches, acoustic/audiovisual strategies, and real-time registration approaches.

AR/VR Approaches. Augmented reality in guidance for surgery is well-investigated with many approaches being presented. We mention here just a few examples to indicate the variety of topics. Liao et al. [372] discuss an AR application for MRI-guided surgery using an animated autostereoscopic image. The integral videography provides geometrically accurate 3D images and reproduces motion parallax without using any supplementary eyeglasses or tracking devices. HoloLens has also been used in recent works for laparoscopic surgery [223] or other ultrasound-guided interventions, such as needle placement [438]. Virtual mirrors as a navigational aid for augmented reality-driven minimally invasive procedures are also encountered in the literature with significant impacts on the accuracy of the procedures [56]. Kalia et al. [282] propose and evaluate a marker-less, intra-operative, AR guidance system for robot-assisted laparoscopic radical prostatectomy. Marker-less approaches were also applied to uterus laparoscopic surgery [113]. Risk assessment and accuracy evaluation have also been conducted in the context of trajectory planning [567] and orthopedic surgery guidance [164]. For breast cancer, AR has been investigated on the basis of 3D ultrasound data [541]. Mixed reality approaches have also been researched [27], and the state of the art is summarized by Kersten-Oertel et al. [297].

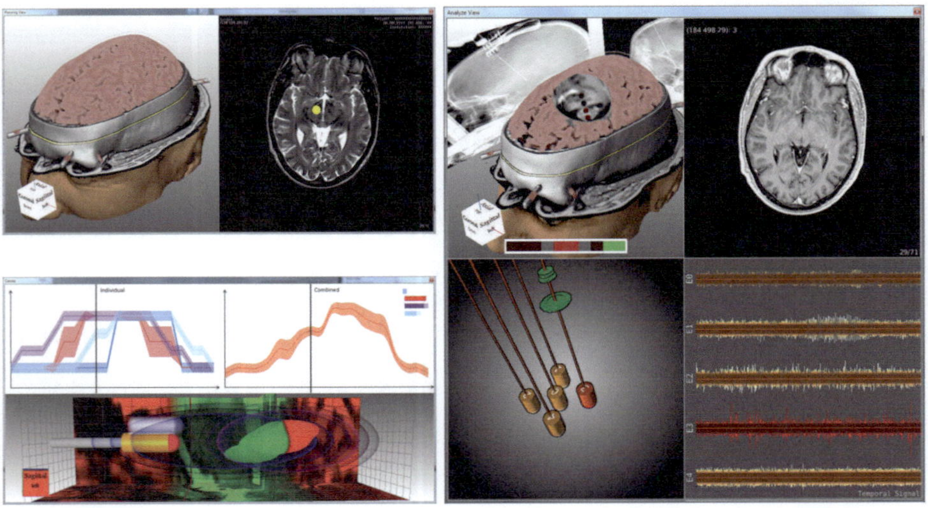

Fig. 3.31 Three supported phases of the system by Bock et al. [64]. Top left: planning, bottom left: placement, right: recording phase (*©2013 IEEE, Reprinted with permission from:* [64])

Multimodal Approaches. Talbot et al. [608] propose the SOFA framework and use it for physically based simulations, with guidance for laparoscopy being an example. They assessed the realism, accuracy, and efficiency of the simulations. Bello et al. [45] developed an integrated system for training visceral needle puncture procedures on the basis of CT data augmented with force measurements in the simulator. Kocev et al. [309] introduced an approach for the simulation of breast biopsy navigation in real time, which integrates information on the soft tissues. Peters et al. [472] discuss a multimodal approach for neurosurgery, where anatomical, vascular, and metabolic data are integrated in a commercially available system. This approach allows the surgeon to obtain an overview of brain structures and to avoid structures of functional significance. Finally, Bock et al. [64] address deep-brain stimulation, which fuses several modalities (imaging data, microelectrode recordings, patient health check-ups, and their respective uncertainties) to support the intra-operative guidance of placing the electrodes (Fig. 3.31).

Acoustic/Audiovisual Approaches. Vetter et al. [642] investigate radio-guided surgery that is additionally supported by the registration of SPECT or PET imaging data. The rapid update of the visual guidance assists the acoustic signal from the radio-guided surgery without slowing down the surgical workflow. Other approaches deal with combining AR with auditory guidance to help resection wound repair, e.g., in nephrectomy [271] and medical needle placement [58]. There are also studies investigating audio-signal guidance in instrument—organ interaction [457]. Improving the 3D perception of an augmented external camera view by combining both auditory and visual stimuli in a dynamic multi-sensory AR environment was investigated by Bork et al. [66].

Registration Approaches. Registration is an indispensable step for guidance in surgery, with a vast corpus of publications. Westermann and Hauser [669] proposed an approach for accurate 3D patient registration to correct movement errors during data acquisition and active patient referencing to update the position of the head during surgery. Registration typically involves various modalities: CT with ultrasound images for liver surgery [293], MRI or CT reconstructions, with the patient's head on the operating table in neurosurgery [200], and also more complex cases such as fluorescence-to-color image alignment for intra-operative augmented reality [498].

3.8.3 Post-operative Assessment

Post-operative assessment includes the evaluation of the accuracy or potential risks from a specific surgical procedure. Rieder et al. [515] proposed a tool to visually support the post-interventional assessment of radiofrequency ablation procedures. Georgii et al. [183] investigated efficient GPU simulation methods for non-invasive tumor treatment using ultrasound therapy. For the oncological assessment in maxillofacial surgery, Pepe et al. [471] combine pattern recognition with mixed reality. Martschinke et al. [395] propose integrated, in-situ surgery planning and assessment tools for breast reconstruction through projection mapping. Training approaches are also proposed, with an example being the work of Stefan et al. [596] for a mixed-reality assessment concept in C-arm-based surgery. The integration of haptics together with visual modalities is also investigated in the work of Mayoral et al. [399] in the context of hip replacement.

> *Most of the approaches in Sect.* 3.8 *deal with* **spatial data** *related to the anatomy of the patient (***organism scale***). The data are mostly* **static** *(for offline approaches)* **or dynamic** *(for in-situ or in-line approaches). As in most cases where medical images are involved, we have* **scalar, low-dimensional data,** *even for multimodal approaches. All methods address the needs of* **practitioners or clinical researchers,** *and they support* **decision-making and communication tasks.**

3.9 Visualization in Educational Contexts

In this section, we discuss visualization approaches that have been employed for biological and/or medical education—either of dedicated personnel, such as nurses and medical students, or the general population, such as schoolchildren. In Fig. 3.32, we see that the topic started early back in the 1980s, but it became very prominent only recently, possibly also with the technological advancements in AR and VR, or the domain of physicalization.

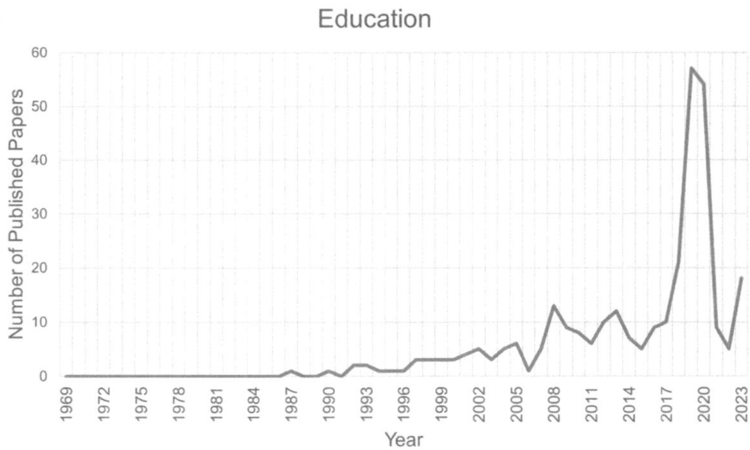

Fig. 3.32 Number of *education and medical training* related papers published over time

3.9.1 Approaches for Biological and Medical Training

Preim and Saalfeld [490] investigated in their survey virtual anatomy education systems, focusing on systems for medical students. Surgical and medical training is one of the traditional applications of visualization and VR/AR technologies, with publications (related to simulators) dating back to 1987 [190]. A significant breakthrough was the work of KARL-HEINZ HÖHNE et al. [241] with their anatomical atlases for volume visualization. Simulations and computer graphics applications targeting teaching surgical operations became popular at the end of the 1990s [77, 131]. This included emerging applications also in VR [86, 660], in combination with haptic interfaces [46] or virtual simulators [65, 131]. These applications encompass a large variety of surgical procedures—from brain surgery to dental surgery and to tumor ablation. They all aim at training medical professionals and allowing them to enhance their skills. Notably, some early applications were targeted at astronauts to prepare them for their missions [423].

In 2004, a paper regarding a knee-joint simulator, accommodating multimodal interactions on phantoms, was published, opening the way for medical education and training in orthopedic surgery [516]. SVAKHINE and colleagues contribute to the state of the art with illustrative visualization approaches for medical training [593, 605]. Another key point was the introduction of GPU accelerations to support the simulation of surgical procedures of complex morphologies, such as the heart [427]. The development of high-quality software volume raycasting systems for large data has also been a driving force for further developments in the field, yielding for instance solutions for illustrative context-enhancing rendering (Fig. 3.33).

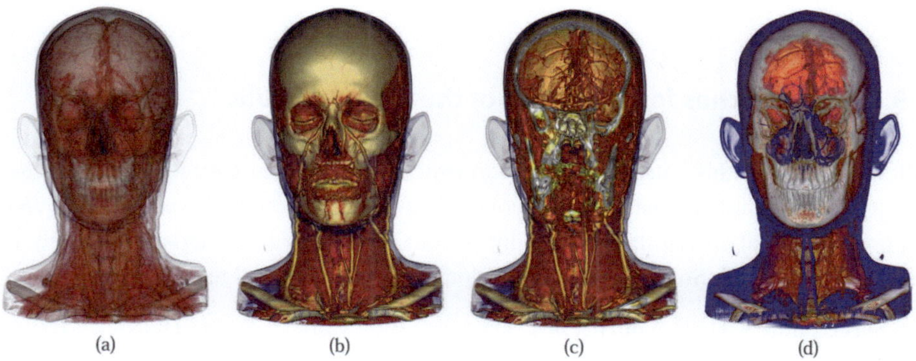

Fig. 3.33 The approach by Bruckner et al. [80] showcased on a contrast-enhanced CT angiography dataset. (a) Gradient-magnitude opacity modulation. (b) Direct volume rendering. (c) Direct volume rendering with cutting plane. (d) Context-preserving illustrative volume rendering. *©2005 The Author(s), Eurographics Proceedings ©2005 The Eurographics Association. Reproduced by kind permission of the Eurographics Association*

Minimally invasive surgery has also been investigated in the context of mixed-reality and VR simulators [35, 341]. AR simulators appeared much later in 2009 and were applied on an ultrasound training scenario [61]. An application that is encountered rarely was an immersive method for collaborative radiological surveying [311].

Several people have contributed in this domain, with the most prominent work being initiated by KUHLEN [628, 629], JOHN [112, 619] and HANSEN [132, 216]. The work of SMIT on the model-based visualization of anatomical data is also a significant contribution [586, 587]. The latter work targets rectal tumor resection and the avoidance of potential damage to nearby structures (Fig. 3.34).

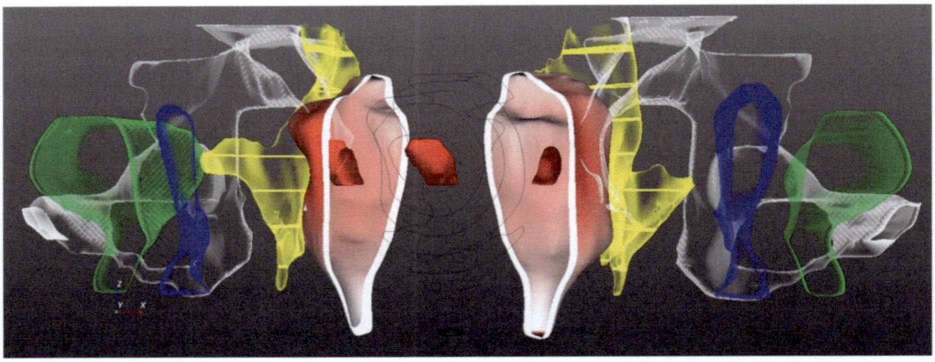

Fig. 3.34 The application of Smit et al. [587] featuring the unfolded 3D model of a female pelvis. *Image courtesy of Noeska Smit, University of Bergen*

3.9.2 Approaches for Education of the General Public

All approaches in this category target the medical or biological education of the general public, such as museum visitors or schoolchildren. They are, therefore, all focusing on the communication of spatial data of low dimensionality; medical data mostly, and only in a few cases biological. Some support the exploration of the data and fewer the analysis.

On-Screen and VR/AR Approaches. The pioneering work of KARL HEINZ HÖHNE and his team is essential. They published a flexible volume model that contained both surface and volume properties of the anatomy and that could be used as an alternative to dissections [241]. A Virtual Reality (VR) approach appeared also shortly after, in 1998 [660]. In this work, Warrick et al. propose a VR strategy based on segmentation and surface rendering that allows students to see the renderings at the same time as the initial medical images. The field continued for many years to introduce contributions mainly in VR.

On-screen approaches started emerging again in the 2000s, probably due to advances in graphics. These spanned from surface and volume visualizations [83, 373, 480, 639] to animations [37]. Popular examples include VOXEL-MAN [480], the open anatomy browser [212], ZygoteBody [63] and the Online Anatomical Human [586]. Furthermore, VR kept growing either with sketch-based approaches, such as the work of Saalfeld et al. [534], or with gaming approaches, such as the VR puzzle proposed by Pohlandt et al. [478] (Fig. 3.35). In AR, mirror approaches also became popular with a notable example being *mirracle* [62].

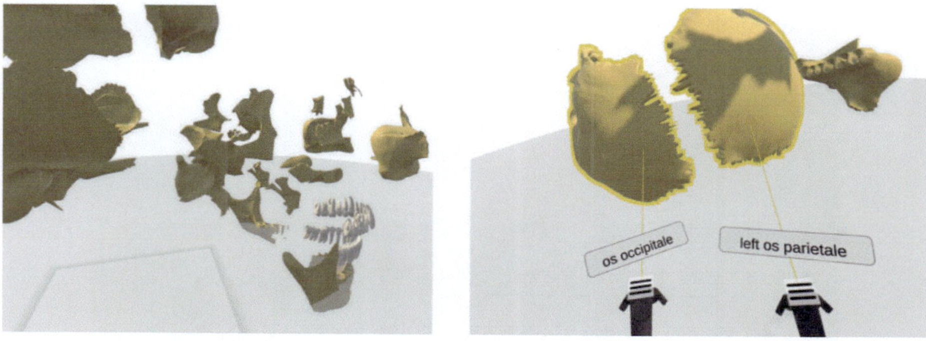

Fig. 3.35 The VR puzzle is embedded in a room, only equipped with a large round ground floor. Pieces are initially distributed. When users select two objects with their controllers, they can start docking them *(From:* [478], *©2019 ACM)*

In this field, there is much less work in the biology domain than in the medical one. Here, learning biomolecular structures has been investigated through gaming in VR [94]. Other approaches focus, for example, on teaching chemistry [161, 607] or biology for STEM education or for K-12 learning [294, 609]. An interesting approach that combines 3D printing with augmented reality was recently presented by Noizet et al. [443]. The most recent work focuses on storytelling approaches to support knowledge discovery about the structure and function of biomolecules [198, 318].

Off-Screen Approaches. Off-screen approaches include fabrication and physicalization of biological and medical data. This has mainly revolved around 3D printing of structures and functions of the human body [19, 337, 506]. Among this, a particular case is the work of Ang et al. [19], who developed a tangible physicalization of cardiac blood flow, to explore 4D MRI data in a slice-based physical model. Medical data physicalizations that do not involve 3D printing are only a few. Recent examples involve the usage of volvelles, which are interactive wheel charts of concentric, rotating disks [599], or computer-generated sliceforms [501]. The former mimics the on-screen fine-tuning of transfer functions to meaningfully display volume data to non-knowledgeable users. The latter proposes a formulation of a volume-based octree to support the partition of space into slices that can be assembled to create a semi-transparent sculpture for anatomy education. Finally, two cases targeting anatomical edutainment are the 2D and 3D *Anatomical Edutainer* [548] (Fig. 3.36) and its subsequent extension to nested papercrafts [547]. The first one targets the generation of 2D printable and 3D foldable physicalizations that change their visual properties (i.e., hues of the visible spectrum) under colored lenses or colored lights, to reveal distinct anatomical structures through user interaction. The second case proposes a new workflow for the computer-aided generation of physicalizations, addressing nested configurations in anatomical and biological structures.

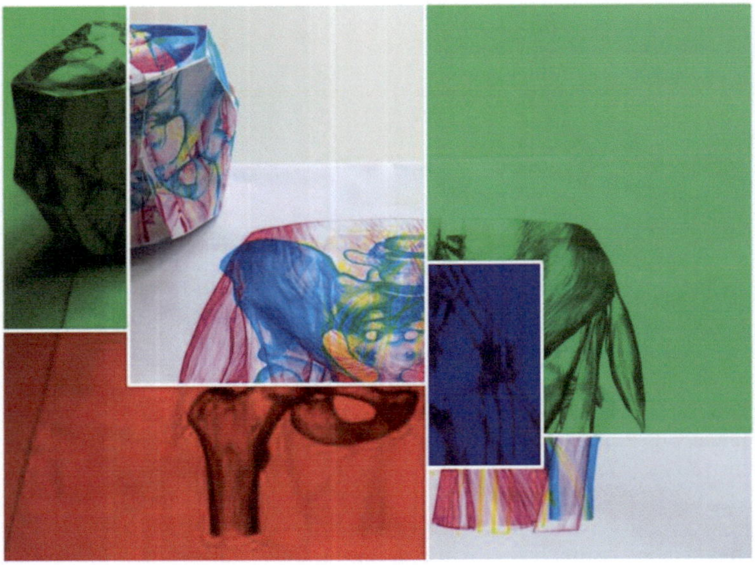

Fig. 3.36 The anatomical edutainer supports 2D printable physicalizations that change their visual properties (i.e., hues of the visible spectrum) under colored lenses, to reveal distinct anatomical structures through user interaction [548]. *Image courtesy of Marwin Schindler, TU Wien*

> *The approaches in Sect.* 3.9 *deal mostly with* ***low-or multi-dimensional spatial data*** *at an* ***organism*** *(MedVis) or* ***molecular*** *(BioVis)* ***scale.*** *The work mostly targets* ***medical students*** *and the* ***general public*** *as users. The work is mostly intended for* ***communication tasks****, but in a few cases also covers data exploration and analysis.*

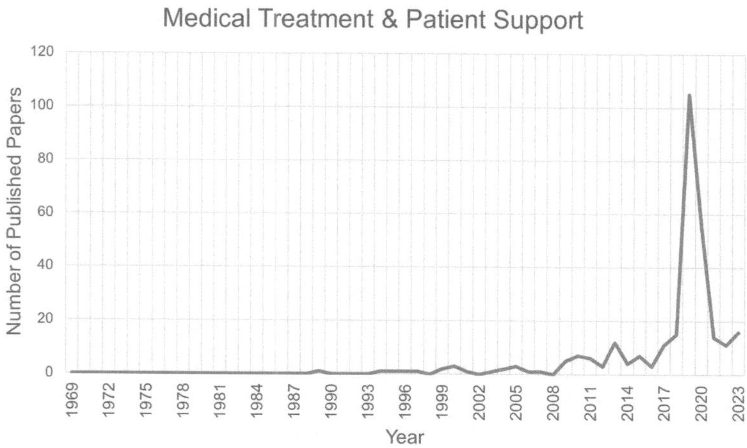

Fig. 3.37 Number of *medical treatment and patient support* related papers published over time

3.10 Visualization for Medical Treatment and Patient Support

In this section, we discuss works in the areas of therapy, rehabilitation, and patient support. The methods presented here frequently involve specialized input devices and adopt modern technologies relatively fast. Subsequently, the majority of the works discussed here are based on mixed-reality environments, where the traditional therapy or rehabilitation approaches are mimicked and enhanced. Figure 3.37 reflects the dependence of these works on available technology. Early works appeared in the 1990s, but we see an increase in the 2010s, when the new generation of mixed-reality devices became accessible. An even bigger recent spike is likely also related to technological advancements, as standalone wireless virtual reality headsets became available around this time.

3.10.1 Psychotherapy

Psychotherapy was one of the first areas where virtual environments (VE) were adopted for patient treatment. The earliest works date back to the 1990s and are focused on exposure and desensitization therapies for anxiety disorders, such as agoraphobia, fear of public speaking, and fear of heights. Here, the idea of adapting traditional approaches to virtual environments is recurrent [444, 530], starting with pioneering work of ROTHBAUM, HODGES, COBLE, and NORTH. Research into the use of VE for psychotherapy has demonstrated certain benefits over traditional therapy techniques such as in-vivo and imaginal therapies. A simulated environment is safe and controlled, can provide fear-producing stimuli for patients that have trouble imagining them, and is more cost-effective by reducing the need to replicate the fear-inducing scenarios in real life. Further, it can be used to identify the particular fear-triggering stimuli by easy repetition of the scenarios. Later, virtual reality (VR) exposure therapy was used to treat addictions [336], as well as post-traumatic stress disorder [520, 529]. Substantial research was also done on the use of VEs for distraction therapy [237] as a treatment for acute and chronic pain. Here, the goal is to achieve a high level of immersion and stimulate the patient's sensory stream with simulated environments, so less attention can be devoted to pain.

The earliest studies on virtual therapy by North et al. [444], as well as many subsequent works, focus on fully immersive virtual environments. Head-mounted displays (HMD) are employed, sometimes combined with additional props or hand-held controllers. However, for a long time, HMDs were affected by technical limitations like low resolution, limited rendering performance, and heavy hardware. This caused patients to experience discomfort and motion sickness, which restricted wider adoption. CAVE-like environments [125] partially addressed these problems, but were expensive and impractical for wider use.

As an alternative, augmented reality (AR) approaches were examined, e.g., marker-based setups and projections [31, 674]. AR approaches were credited with a greater sense of presence for patients and a more natural patient-therapist interaction. They shared the same augmented space and the therapist could easily observe the patient's behavior. However, the early approaches also required complicated setups, e.g., cameras, markers, large displays, or projectors.

Most of the VE-based therapeutic systems from the 1990s were just prototypes and proofs of concept. Around the turn of the century first dedicated commercialized solutions began to appear, e.g., Virtually Better [236]. The research gained momentum in the 2010s, supported by the availability of off-the-shelf technologies, such as the NINTENDO WII and a new generation of HMDs. New application examples include diagnostics and treatment of ADHD (attention deficit hyperactivity disorder) [3] and cognitive and autism-spectrum disorders, including behavioral therapy and social skills training [284]. Gamification was also integrated into virtual environments to increase a patient's engagement in the treatment. For instance, a game is based on holding eye contact with a virtual avatar for social training of autistic children [499]. Such applications have been referred to as *serious games*.

Another recent trend is treatment personalization, which is supported by the availability of mobile devices. Therapists can provide patients with a set of exercises to be executed at home, monitor their progress, and adjust the difficulty level. For example, the VR acrophobia treatment introduced by Wagner et al. [651] offers scenarios of various difficulties (Fig. 3.38). Similarly, Lindner et al. [376] employ different levels of realism in their serious game for arachnophobia treatment. Finally, several self-guided approaches have been proposed, intended for personal use without a therapist's supervision. Typical representatives are mobile applications or VR games for relaxation and stress management, where visual depictions and virtual environments guide users through calming exercises [512].

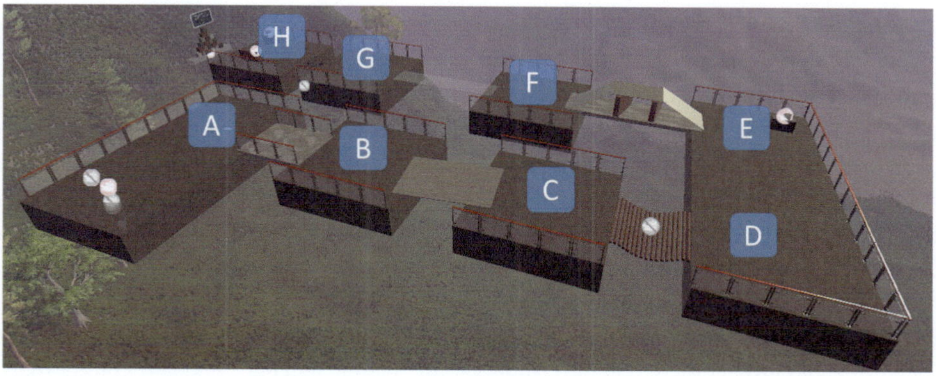

Fig. 3.38 A bridge scenario in VR acrophobia treatment with locations of varying difficulty, such as solid or unstable ground, with or without railing [651]. *©2020 The Author(s), Eurographics Proceedings ©2020 The Eurographics Association. Reproduced by kind permission of the Eurographics Association*

3.10.2 Rehabilitation

In the area of rehabilitation, we can observe similar patterns and a similar timeline concerning VE adoption to those in psychotherapy. However, VE-based physical rehabilitation is even more intertwined with technological developments. From the very beginning, VE rehabilitation systems were typically paired with various input devices for motion tracking such as haptic gloves or marker-based trackers to enable the measurement of a patient's performance. Haptic-feedback devices, such as the Phantom [396], were (and still are) utilized for hand rehabilitation and motor-skill training. Later, EEG and EMG trackers were employed to get further data on a patient's functioning. Initially, a significant portion of computer-assisted rehabilitation research focused on the development of new technologies and devices. In 2010 well-performing commercial VR and AR technologies, e.g., Kinect or LeapMotion, became widely available, and VE-based therapy and rehabilitation started moving from "the technology development focus, to one that focuses on how (already available) technology can support rehabilitation principles and outcomes." [664]

We differentiate between two types of rehabilitation targets—cognitive and motor skills. Both are particularly important for post-stroke patient rehabilitation, which was one of the first areas, where VEs were applied. The goal is to improve the patient's activities of daily living. Initial approaches focused on motor-skill rehabilitation, predominantly for upper extremities (e.g., reaching tasks, grip training, hand-eye coordination). They typically combined haptic devices with on-screen task representations [242, 482], which were later replaced by augmented reality and fully immersive environments. Different visual/virtual representations were studied for three main tasks: (1) providing instructions—task demonstrations, patterns to trace, or visual cues during task performance, (2) motivating the patients—using gamification and metaphors with common tasks, and (3) providing feedback on patients' performance—for example, visual error augmentation [531] was studied as a mean to improve the patients' performance.

VEs were also used as a substitute for traditional mirror therapy [386], where a patient observes the motion of a healthy limb in place of the affected one, providing the illusion of normal movement. A similar concept is employed to treat phantom pains for amputees. Another area of motor rehabilitation is gait analysis. Here, VE devices are typically paired with treadmill devices and present balance-training tasks, such as stepping over virtual obstacles [259]. VEs also motivate patients to walk by providing nice environments that can be explored and by incorporating gamification elements [296]. Visual cues on step placement were also examined [262]. Recent works in gait analytics include KAVAGait [650], a system for storing and inspection of complex, time-varying patient gait data, and gaitXplorer [650], an explainability-enriched visual analytics approach for the classification of gait patterns.

Regarding cognitive skills, e.g., in post-stroke, dementia, or brain injury patients, VEs are used both for diagnosis and assessment as well as for rehabilitation [441]. VEs typically simulate daily tasks such as grocery shopping or crossing the road [652]. This includes tasks to target specific cognitive domains, such as attention, concentration, memory, and spatial awareness [647]. VEs also play an important role in prosthetic [442, 475] and wheelchair [23] training, where they are employed to accustom the patient to a prosthesis or wheelchair, respectively.

3.10.3 Patient Support

In the past ten years we have seen an emergence of visualization research focused on patient support, patient-clinician communication, and personalized healthcare. Extended reality applications have been examined to facilitate telepresence for rehabilitation [171], but also for patient support and remote health consultations [299, 686]. In the domain of telemedicine, we find visualization dashboards and visual analytics applications dedicated to remote health monitoring, e.g., reports from smart wearables or home sensors [186] that inform caregivers of the current patient status or notify them of a medical emergency. Besides sensor-based reporting, applications have been designed to aid patients in reporting their own experiences and symptoms. For example, Hong et al.'s [247] Visual Observations of Daily Living help pediatric patients with chronic diseases to report their daily experiences through a library of symptom illustrations.

In recent years wearable devices and tracking of personal health-related data have become common. Tracked data typically include a number of daily steps, heart rate, sleep stages, as well as activity types or food consumption that users log themselves. This led to the research of visualizations to support the exploration and sense-making of personal data for audiences without medical education beyond standard overviews provided by a plethora of available tracking applications. SleepExplorer [371] enables users to find correlations between their sleep quality and daily activity. Caballero et al. [173] introduce V-Awake, a

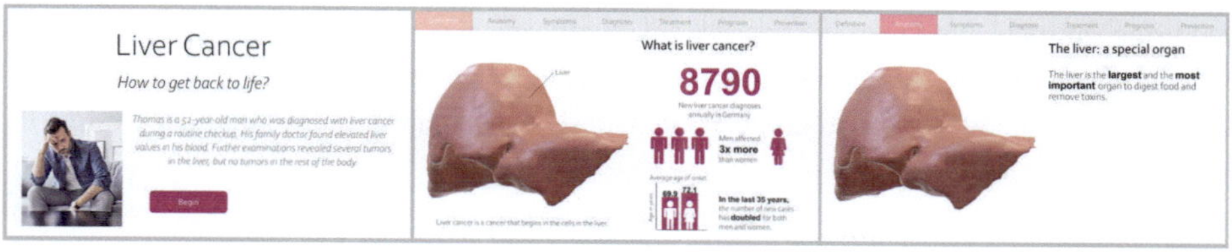

Fig. 3.39 An excerpt from a liver cancer story designed for patients and general public education. *Reprinted from [402], ©2022, with permission from Elsevier Ltd.*

visual analytics approach that aids users to find, store, analyze, and correct sleep staging outcomes from deep-learning models, in the absence of ground truth. Their subsequent work, PerSleep [92], supports further explainability of the deep-learning models, focusing on understanding their performance. Other works, such as DataSelfie [300] and Trackly [26] explore the customizable design for personal data visualization to increase user agency.

Visualizations have been also utilized for patient education. There are cases of AR and VR applications, such as tours of operating theaters to minimize a patient's anxiety [463], illustrations and animations explaining disease concepts or treatment procedures employing various anatomical representations [486]. Also narrative visualizations are combined with multiple modalities and narrative commentaries to educate patients and the broader audience about a disease, associated risks, or medical procedures [74, 208, 402]. Visualizations for patient education and communication, particularly narrative visualizations, have not yet been thoroughly explored and present one of the open challenges in medical visualization [191]. An early example of a narrative visualization in a medical context is given in Fig. 3.39. More recent work on narrative visualization addresses the role of characters, in particular individual patients and physicians that allow viewers to sympathize and connect to these protagonists [88, 416]. Such a personal connection may potentially improve engagement and consequently compliance of patients. However, the current research is far from allowing definitive conclusions.

> *The approaches in Sect.* 3.10 *deal mostly with* ***low- or multi-dimensional spatial and abstract data*** *at an* ***organism scale.*** *The work targets* ***researchers, practitioners, and patients*** *as users. Initially, the work focused on* ***communication tasks,*** *then evolved to cover also* ***exploration and analysis.***

3.11 Visualization of Electronic Health Records

In clinical practice, patient health records are composed of multivariate and multi-dimensional data, containing image data (e.g., CT scans, MRIs), tabular data (e.g., blood and urine samples), and textual reports (e.g., symptoms reported by the patient). All records have temporal stamps and an important chronological order. This poses a significant challenge for the management and analysis of such data, especially under time constraints that clinicians often face.

In Fig. 3.40, we see that the topic dates back to the 1990s, but it started becoming more prominent recently, potentially due to the COVID-19 pandemic and also due to the development of solutions that handle more robustly big heterogeneous data sets. A pioneering work in the visualization of patient histories was LifeLines by CATHERINE PLAISANT and BEN SHNEIDERMAN [477]. LifeLines (Fig. 3.41) enabled the visualization of various medical events and data such as diagnoses, prescriptions, lab results, and imaging data on a timescale using color and line thickness encodings. Initially, the system was designed for the visualization of a single patient history. Later it was extended to cover records of multiple patients, providing options for the temporal alignment of records based on the events in the data (e.g., admission into hospital or symptom onset) [658]. Later works built on the LifeLines concept with additional techniques to filter, align, and aggregate medical event-based records [422, 672]. They provided insight into disease progression patterns, typical patient flows between hospital departments, or monitoring data from an intensive care unit.

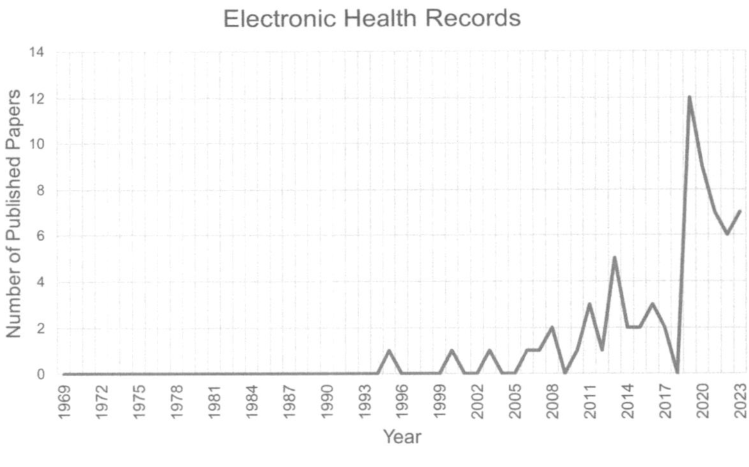

Fig. 3.40 Number of *electronic health records* visualization papers published over time

Following systems focusing on the general representation of patient histories, there is an emergence of cohort-based approaches. They use health-record visualization for specific applications such as the assessment of treatment plans [8, 201], characterization of a given disease, and prediction of outcomes for the patient. Notable works can be found particularly in the area of cancer treatment in Sect. 3.5.3.

Many of the previously mentioned systems relied on well-structured data, e.g., explicit lists of symptoms and predefined disease categorization. However, medical records often

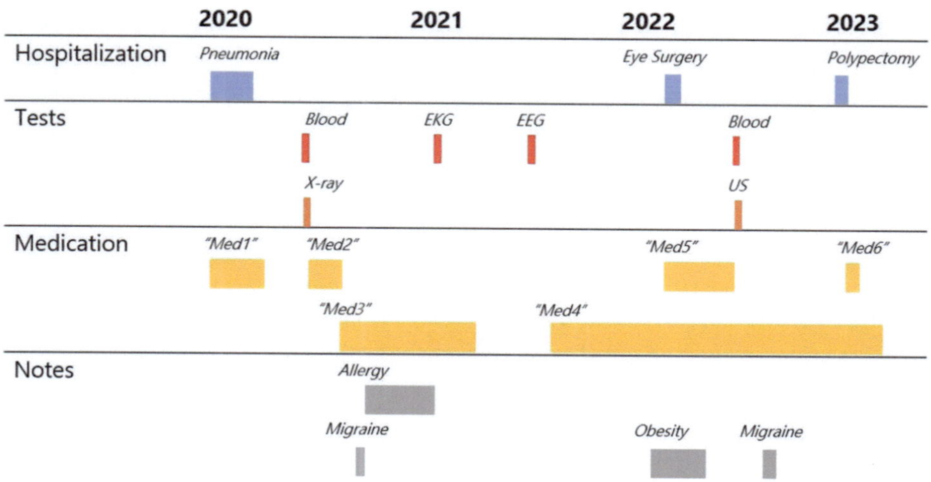

Fig. 3.41 The patient history over several years is summarized based on events, categorized, e.g., in tests and hospitalizations. Easily distinguishable colors are used for the presentation of each category. *Image inspired by the work of Plaisant et al.* [477]

come as unstructured texts. In recent years, machine learning (ML) and natural language processing (NLP) have been combined with visualization to address this problem. Notably, Sultanum et al. [603] presented Doccurate, an NLP-based approach for the creation of user-curated views of patient history from textual notes. ML is nowadays applied to electronic health records (EHRs) to extract information and also to provide clinical decision support, e.g., by risk prediction or treatment plan suggestion. Several visual analytics approaches, such as RetainVis by Kwon et al. [340] and CarePre by Jin et al. [270], have been proposed to support the explainability of and insight into ML decisions. Recent trends in EHR visualization have been summarized by Wang and Laramee [657].

> *The approaches in Sect.* 3.11 *deal with* ***high-dimensional and temporal data*** *and with scenarios at an* ***organism and group scale.*** *The work targets* ***practitioners, researchers, and patients*** *as users. The work covers the* ***whole spectrum of tasks.***

3.12 Visualization for Public Health and Epidemiology

Most research in medical data analysis and visualization, for example in the Visual Analytics in Healthcare (VAHC) workshop series, tackles *clinical* medicine, i.e., the diagnosis and treatment of individual patients. *Public health* (PH), in contrast, aims at understanding health indicators at a population level and ultimately at *preventing* diseases.

PH authorities at regional, national, and international levels—with the World Health Organization on top—collect data to monitor the health status of populations. For prevention, it is essential to monitor the changing incidence of diseases and also to analyze health indicators, such as the amount of obesity, smoking, or alcohol drinking in a population. Experts with different backgrounds, e.g., in medicine, statistics, and health economy, cooperate to analyze data and communicate the findings to inform health-policy decision-makers.

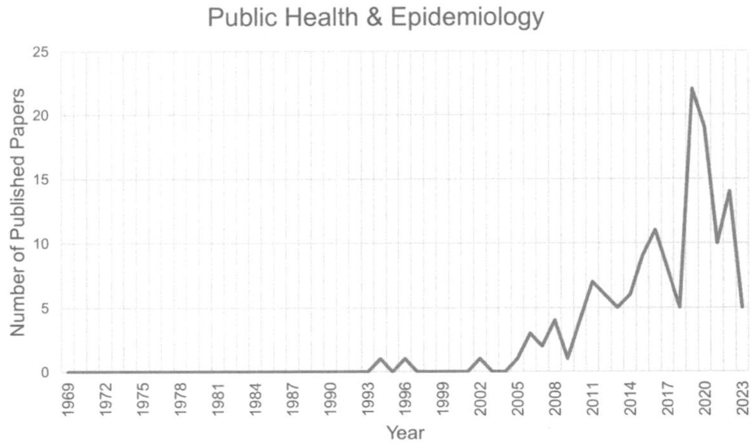

Fig. 3.42 Number of *public health and epidemiology* related papers published over time

Visual analytics can strongly contribute to the sense-making process related to these large, high-dimensional, and spatio-temporal data [454, 485, 561]. In Fig. 3.42, we see that the topic started around 2008 when the large population studies started and evolved [485] recently, partially due to the COVID-19 pandemic. The essential spatial character of the data led to the development of *health geography*. Cartography experts employ and adapt their techniques to convey spatial health-related information. They identify disease clusters and also correlate the local load of diseases with the availability of specialized hospitals. As a pioneer of cartography visualization, McEachren made a number of contributions to public health [101, 521]. An essential aspect is to perform the analysis at different scales, since very local characteristics may influence the likelihood of diseases. More specifically, *choropleth maps*, where attributes are color-coded for administrative units, are frequently used to convey the incidence of diseases. The discrete character of this map type is sometimes inappropriate which leads to the use of heatmaps instead.

3.12.1 Cohort Studies

To analyze the health status of a population and its development over time, cohort studies are carried out. A random sample of a defined population, e.g., a county, is examined regularly, e.g., in five-year intervals. Huge amounts of data are acquired for all participants, covering information from urine and blood samples, many other diagnostic tests, answers from interviews, and medical imaging data. The major goal of the expensive examinations is to identify and characterize risk factors for the outbreak of a disease, or an early and severe outbreak of a disease. A special focus lies on *preventable risk factors*. Visual analytics can support this reasoning process. Klemm et al. [305] combined information derived from MRI data, e.g., the shape of the spine, with socio-demographic data, such as sleeping behavior, to understand how back pain arises (Fig. 3.43).

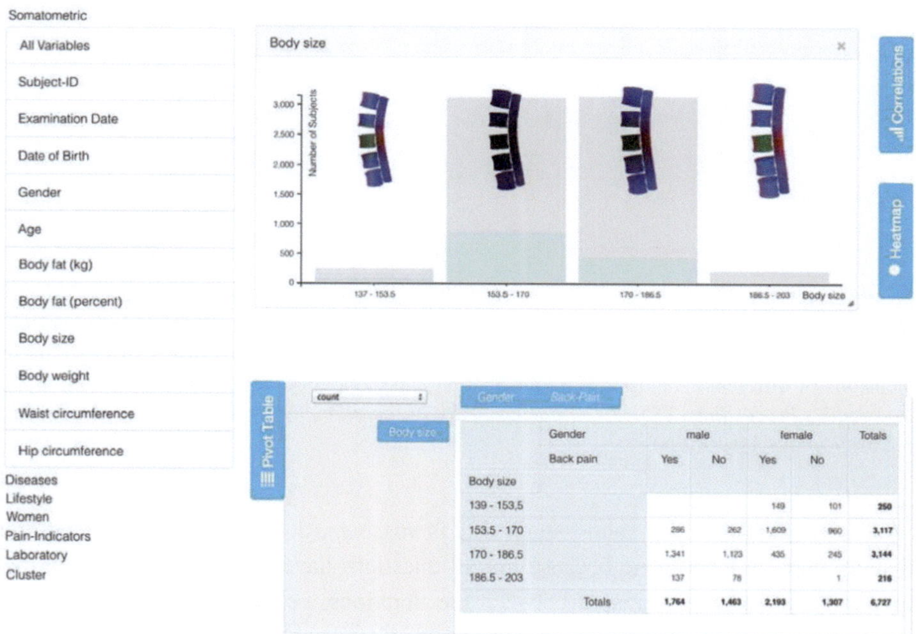

Fig. 3.43 Visual analytics for heterogeneous cohort data, where spine shape is correlated with other patient variables, e.g., gender, height, and pain (*©2014 IEEE, Reprinted with permission from:* [305])

Klemm et al. [304] addressed the problem of efficiently finding strong correlations among a large number of attributes. First, they efficiently computed correlations through extensive parallelization. The results were presented in *regression cubes*. The combined influence of two potential risk factors such as increased weight and alcohol consumption on disease incidence could be characterized. While strong correlations may be due to a causal relation, this is not always the case. More support is necessary to identify causal relations efficiently. Alemzadeh et al. [14] made another attempt to characterize subpopulations with an increased risk for a health disorder, such as a fatty liver. They performed subspace clustering, guided by a few constraints specified by the experts. A comprehensive visual exploration of the clustering results is provided (Fig. 3.44).

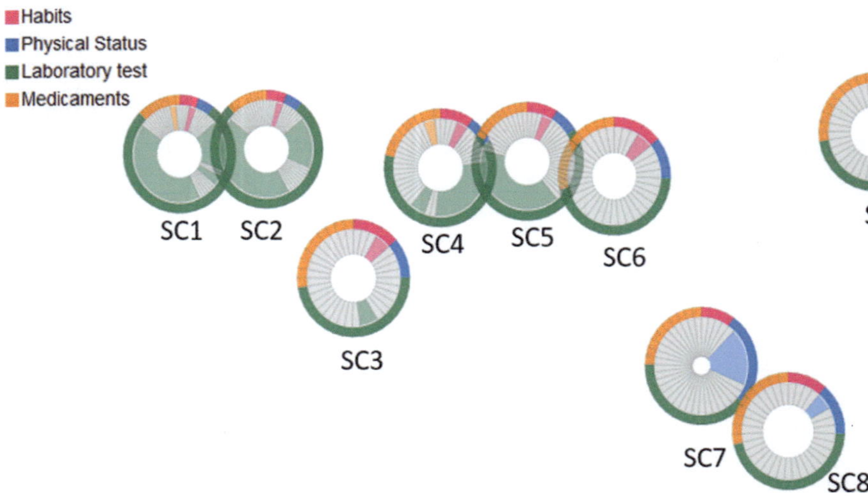

Fig. 3.44 Overview of the subspace clusters of a cohort-study data [14]. Subspace clusters are shown as donuts where elements with a larger inner circle (hole) represent clusters with few members. Gray values represent dimensions that do not contribute to a specific subspace cluster. Colors represent dimensions of different categories, e.g., medication and laboratory values. *©2017 The Author(s), Eurographics Proceedings ©2017 The Eurographics Association. Reproduced by kind permission of the Eurographics Association*

An essential problem in cohort-study data is *missingness*. Data within one iteration of the study may be incomplete because not all questions have been answered. Even more importantly, there is missingness between the iterations, i.e., participants may drop out for various reasons. Alemzadeh et al. [15] provide a display of the missingness patterns and imputation strategies that aim at replacing missing values in case their absence is not completely random.

3.12.2 Outbreak Detection and Surveillance

It is essential to detect outbreaks of diseases, primarily infectious diseases, but also food-borne or water-borne diseases. If an outbreak has been detected, it needs to be monitored, and predictions are required to support health policies. As in the COVID-19 pandemic, there can be strong dynamics that lead to a high urgency in deciding on effective measures.

Again, visual analytics contributes to outbreak detection and an analysis of the effects of potential countermeasures. Simulation models predict the further course of a pandemic. The parameters of these models are continuously adapted based on real development. Pioneering work was carried out by MACIEJEWSKI and EBERT. They developed techniques to identify syndromic hotspots [392] and to model and visualize the course of a pandemic [391].

The COVID-19 pandemic also triggered research activities in outbreak detection and surveillance. Many concepts and techniques that were earlier developed for analyzing pandemic influenza waves could be reused [6]. Afzal et al. [5] modeled and visualized the course of the pandemic, but they also considered the availability of resources, such as hospital beds and places in intensive care units, to provide better decision support. Leung et al. [363] applied frequent item mining to understand chains of and reasons for infections as a basis for visualizations. Such methods can provide deeper insights into situations that lead to infections.

> *The approaches in Sect.* 3.12 *deal with* ***spatial and abstract high-dimensional and temporal data.*** *PH addresses challenges at a* ***group scale,*** *dealing with cohorts and populations. The work targets* ***researchers, decision-makers, patients, and the general public*** *as users. It is intended for* ***analysis, decision-making, and communication tasks.***

4 Position Statements

For a broader perspective on the evolution of the BioMedVis field, we contacted more than 50 researchers of mixed seniority and expertise, both from industry and academia and from all around the world. The intention was to have an overview of the status of the domain—not only from the point of published literature but also from the people forming the field. We collected answers in written form from 16 participants, whose characteristics can be seen in Table 4.1. Below, we summarize the responses that we obtained from the participants, per question and anonymized—as requested by them.

Table 4.1 The background and characteristics of the 16 researchers participating in our interview

Participant	A	B	C	D	E	F	G	H	I	J	K	L	M	N	O	P
Seniority 1 = Junior 3 = Senior	3	2	2	3	3	3	3	1	1	3	3	2	1	2	3	3
Expertise Bio Med	Bio	Bio	Bio Med	Bio	Med	Bio	Bio Med	Med	Med	Med	Bio Med	Med	Bio	Bio	Med	Bio
Gender	m	m	f	m	f	f	m	m	m	m	m	m	f	m	m	m
Background Academia Industry	Academia	Academia Industry	Academia	Academia	Academia	Academia	Academia	Academia	Academia	Academia	Academia	Academia Industry	Academia	Academia	Academia	Academia

K. Furmanová et al., *BioMedical Visualization*, Synthesis Lectures on Visualization,
https://doi.org/10.1007/978-3-031-66789-3_4

4.1 Interviews

Q1: In your view, when was the "golden age" of BioMedVis? Is it still lasting?

The answers to this question revolve around three-time frames. The first group of participants (5 people) considers that the golden age of the field was around the years 2000–2010, the second group considered the timeframe between 1980 and 2000 (3 people, the most senior among our participants), and the third group (8 people, mostly junior researchers) expressed that the golden age is still to come. For example, participant **L** commented "I don't think we have reached it yet. [...] In 2000–2010, BioMedVis had a lot of attention [...] But then again, I see surprisingly little impact from those academic achievements in terms of what healthcare is using today". Among all answers, four participants (of varying expertise and seniority) see a difference between the golden age of MedVis and BioVis: "MedVis had some golden age, maybe around the turn of the century, or also a few years thereafter; I'm still waiting for the golden age of BioVis, I'd say, even though clearly lots of very good works were published already" (participant **G**). Also, three participants mentioned a shift in topics "from the lower hanging fruits to more complex, larger datasets and application areas" (participant **H**) and that research "was more driven by algorithm development than it is today" (participant **A**).

Q2: What problems are you considering as solved in BioMedVis?

Regarding solved problems, most of the participants comment about volume visualization (indirect and direct) for small, single-modality datasets (8 people). A few more participants extended this to all kinds of basic visualization or data representations (4 people). Other topics that emerged in the answers were related to "genome browsing; visualization of transcriptomic/proteomic data; visualization of microscopic neuronal circuits of moderate size" (participant **K**). However, most of the interviewees do not see volume rendering as a completely solved issue. In many cases, even topics that are seemingly solved can benefit or have benefited from improvements. For example, participant **C** commented that "many problems in MedVis (and some in BioVis) are sufficiently solved, so that applications can build upon them satisfyingly; while, of course, one can always argue that some further improvements always are possible." Participant **J** mentioned that "[fields] such as direct volume rendering or isosurface extraction got quite an impact by getting deep-learning methods involved," which indicates that there is a constant evolution of many major topics in BioMedVis.

Q3: Has BioMedVis changed during the years you are in the field? If yes, how?

Unanimously the participants agreed that the field has faced many changes. As succinctly put by one of the most senior participants: "having been in the field for over 40 years, everything has changed: computing, graphics, and data" (participant **D**). Some identified a change in topics: "Quite a few sub-topics in BioMedVis have transitioned towards the right along Gartner's hype cycle (from a pioneering stage, to a hype stage, [and] to a maturing stage)" (participant **G**). Others saw a change in the nature of the research—going from exploratory to quantitative visualization: "where users can extract hard numbers, not just general ideas or vague trends" (participant **H**), in data complexity and size: "There were only some first datasets (like gene expression data) out there, which is nothing compared to the different omics data we have nowadays [...]" (participant **J**), public dataset availability: "20 or 30 years ago it was even difficult to get a single CT of a patient," (participant **N**), and in scope—now moving across many more scales and more modalities, and opening more computational possibilities. Also, the accompanying or enabling technologies have changed, e.g., "when WebGL started to become popular [... and ...] was available on all browsers and then later on smartphones. This really pushed accessible BioMedVis" (participant **I**). A participant commented on the nature of contributions that we see: they revolve more around "systems and larger, combined datasets" (participant **P**), meaning that there has been a "transition from a stronger algorithmic focus to a more application focus [...] This has benefits, as people visualize relevant real-world data instead of only a few toy data sets, but also comes with the downside of being less generalizable [...]" (participant **A**). This also indicates a movement "towards more and more complex problems that can only be solved when bringing together expertise from different areas" (participant **E**), which seems to have been facilitated also by "the advent of Data Science, [...while...] the (renewed) rise of AI has opened up new avenues for the application of Machine Learning (deep or not) in biology and medicine" (participant **K**).

Q4: Are you considering BioVis and MedVis as tightly related or rather separate research fields, and why?

Although it has been stated by several interviewees that "the overall goal is to have a comprehensive look at patients over multiple scales ranging from organs to cells to genes and beyond" (participant **J**), most of them agree that the two fields remain quite detached from each other. Few (mostly those coming from BioVis) consider the fields "tightly related. Not always, but there are definitely problems where both fields play a role and need to work together" (participant **B**). There are many reasons for that: one participant commented that "BioVis has so far been more InfoVis and MedVis more SciVis (though there are exceptions and probably different ideas on where to draw the boundaries)" (participant **L**), while another commented that "BioVis can be characterized as exploratory visualization, while MedVis also needs explanatory visualization" (participant **O**). Most people see or wish for more collaboration and tight integration of the two fields: "If we'd follow what is needed and what makes sense, both fields would do more to grow together and help each other" (participant **G**) and they give as an example of interrelation the application of "omics" techniques in medicine (participant **K**). There are, though, several obstacles for this. For instance, "there is an important distinction based on end-user characteristics" (participant **L**).

Q5: Do you think BioMedVis is an exciting and important research domain? Why?

All interviewees agreed on the field being both exciting and important. "It is exciting because of the complexity of the systems under study, and the need for clear visual representations and models to aid in their understanding, analysis, and application. It is important because it pertains to our understanding of ourselves and our health and well-being" (participant **D**). Also, many participants see "so many challenges [to address], including physiology, cohorts, systems questions [...] and outstanding options for impact, e.g., relating to P4 (or P5) medicine" (participant **G**). Others have mentioned interpretability: "There are enormous efforts in AI-based medical image analysis, but with much less impact than one would think and hope, and one reason is poor understanding of the visualization piece" (participant **L**). The reliability of data analysis, where visualization can contribute a lot was, also brought up (participant **E**). One participant (**P**) noticed "that the education and communication about both topics [i.e., Medicine and Biology] are essential, and here visualization can also contribute to a large degree."

Q6: Mention the two most significant past achievements of BioMedVis. What makes them significant?

As for the major accomplishments in the areas, most participants said it was hard to pick just two of all the important work that has been done over the years. However, several of them did not hesitate to mention specific papers or working groups in connection to significant work (either important to the community or personally to their own work).

Most of the participants comment in some way on volume rendering—direct or indirect—as being one of the most significant achievements of the field: "Going all the way back in time, volume visualization was a major improvement in the medical field for getting insight into imaging data" (participant **J**). One participant pointed out: "Given that such solutions are by now standard and really widespread in products everywhere in medicine, where 3D data is acquired, quite clearly documents their significance" (participant **G**). In connection to this, the Marching Cubes paper [385] was singled out by at least four participants as being a very influential piece of work: "Marching Cubes paved the way for robust extraction of isosurfaces from a volume, in spite of ambiguity issues" (participant **O**).

In MedVis, visualization of blood flow in combination with volume rendering was mentioned as well: "[...] because it has found its way to clinical application, often because it was developed in collaboration with medical scientists or clinicians" (participant **K**). Reformation techniques were also mentioned by two participants, focusing on flattening for colonoscopy (participants **G** and **O**) or curved planar reformation for angiography (participant **G**). Here, "simple MPR views" have been particularly credited (participant **H**) due to their widespread use. Other topics mentioned are web-based visualizations (participant **I**).

In BioVis, one participant highlighted "the use of biological molecular visualization for the design of novel biomedical therapeutics" (participant **D**). More often, omics-related approaches in the context of biological function and diagnostics are highlighted here. For example, participant **F** commented that a significant achievement is "Genome Browsers, [as] everyone uses them all the time," while participant **K** focuses on the use of network visualization for pathways or neuronal circuits. In the same context, Circos [330] was also mentioned, which "made a tremendous number of magazine covers, and thus gave terrific publicity to data visualization, despite its patent and acknowledged legibility shortcomings" (participant **C**).

Q7: Mention the two most significant current trends in BioMedVis. What makes them significant?

Concerning current trends in the field, almost all participants highlighted the use or integration of visualization solutions with machine learning and (explainable) artificial intelligence. This also relates, as many of them commented, to the trend of going from "individual data sets to collections, such as cohorts" (participant **J**) or the "huge increase in data sizes" (participant **F**) and "the increasing scale and complexity at which data have to be handled" (participant **K**). In the context of data complexity, participant **H** highlights two specific applications: the visualization of high-resolution neuronal datasets for connectomics, and visual analysis tools for immunofluorescence imaging and high-throughput screening.

"Applied deep learning for more thorough examination and complex diagnosis" is also mentioned (participant **O**), while "the application of data science and AI techniques [...] leads to an increasing need for close collaboration between computer scientists and people from the biological or medical domain" (participant **K**). This trend is encountered both in the medical and the biological subdomain, and in the latter, it is often indicated in conjunction with single-cell data, whole genome sequencing, or multi-omics applications—also linking to personalized treatment (participants **N** and **J**) or finding new biomarkers (participant **A**).

With regard to biological applications, "bridging bio-computation and visualization" was also referred to, as "it makes data visualization an integral component of the scientific discovery loop, as opposed to an after-process" (participant **C**). Many participants stressed also the importance of explainable AI: "However, one substantial challenge is often the interpretation of the machine learning methods, which can be addressed with visualization" (participant **F**). Interestingly, some participants also see the need for collaborative visualization: "[...] big problems that require multiple experts looking at the data at the same time" (participant **C**), for reliable automation (participant **E**), for web-based visualizations (**I**), and for bigger tools and toolkits: "[...] more relevant in practice but more difficult for smaller groups and single PhD students to be successful" (participant **P**). Two participants also indicated VR and AR, e.g., in the context of "XR-based operations [...which are...] expected to outperform the traditional operation style" (participant **O**). However one of them commented that "[they] have a lot of influence [...]; significance: not sure, we will see" (participant **P**).

Q8: Mention the two most significant open challenges in BioMedVis. Why are you considering them as open problems? What would be required to solve these problems?

Regarding the open challenges, there was a bigger variety in the responses—potentially triggered by the research interests and directions that our participants pursue. One open challenge, as prominently expressed by several participants, is the combination of AI together with visualization, especially with regard to healthcare decision-making support. As participant **L** stated this is a matter of data: "The core of this challenge is the actual situation for decisions in healthcare: messy, high time-pressure, much data but unclear what's relevant, etc." Yet, participant **G** generalizes it to a better integration "with the computational world (machine learning, statistics, data science)." As mentioned by participant **F**, "intelligent and good aggregation methods is for me an open challenge" as current approaches, e.g., for dimensionality reduction, no longer suffice. Explainable AI is also a recurring topic: "Another open challenge is to make full use of deep-learning techniques in a transparent way. Here, the analysis process can presumably benefit substantially from deep-learning solutions, but the details are not always worked out yet and the process needs to be transparent" (participant **J**).

Another challenge that was brought up by several people relates to bridging scales: "We know very well how to visualize microscopic neuronal circuits on the one hand, and macroscopic anatomical and functional structures on the other by (f)MRI or PET, but bridging the gap is still an unsolved problem" (participant **K**). This could be within the context of integrated diagnostics: "How do we combine imaging (radiology, pathology) with molecular analysis from genomics and proteomics?" (participant **L**). Bridging the scales is also challenging due to magnitude differences between scales: "The challenge is that the scales are [different] by an order of magnitude that does not allow you to register data automatically or to relate the different scales to each other without further knowledge" (participant **J**). This challenge includes phenomena across a wide range of scales—both spatial and temporal: "One thing that would be needed are modeling tools that seamlessly enable interactive simulation with visualization with real-time "handshaking" between levels of theory and complexity" (participant **D**). Participant **N** remarked on full-body visualization: "Capture, analyze and visualize the full body of a person. Well, there is no system that allows us to analyze a full dataset of a person with enough resolution, enough variables."

A third challenge relates to the actual implementation of visualizations and visual interfaces. This came up in three different contexts: as a need to "provide a reusable software platform to address different BioMedVis applications: a lot of time goes into system development" (participant **P**), to support reusability: "Define a key toolbox of visual elements, stop reinventing chart types with new names in each subdiscipline" (participant **M**), and to simplify workflows and create sustainable tools and libraries: "Tools and libraries are often not well supported and have no active community contributing to them. That's why many groups need to reinvent the wheel over and over again" (participant **B**).

Personalization and democratization of BioMedical visualizations were also pointed out: "[...] personal visualizations of BioMed data that are easily accessible and affordable, for example for low-income societies" (participant **K**), web-based visualization: "Web-based real-time rendering of extremely large datasets" (participant **I**), or instant molecular simulations: "Being able to test in a few seconds at most, a single drug, would ease the generation of vaccines, and other kinds of treatments" (participant **N**). Confidence and uncertainty were also discussed: "Everything related to reliability, robustness, uncertainty is a big challenge. This entails quantification and communication about these aspects" (participant **E**).

Q9: Do you see any new application domains for BioMedVis in the future?

Many interviewees discuss topics that bridge BioVis and MedVis—for example, "simultaneous visualizations of imaging and omics data" (participant **F**). Genomics and —omics, in general, are mentioned several times, as "visualization method to support these complex analyses [i.e., for large panels for all cancers in healthcare] does not exist yet" (participant **L**). Other popular topics concern new visualizations for communicating complex biological phenomena, for mass communication, e.g., within the context of pandemics, for communicating a health status and treatment plan to a patient, or for communicating personal data using "a significantly larger scale of personal health data" (participant **G**). As new data acquisition techniques appear, several interviewees commented that there will be a need for new image and volume data visualization, interpretation, and integration tools. Other emerging topics include synthetic biology, population biology, epidemiology, precision medicine, biomedical issues related to climate change, computational forensics, and cultural anthropology. Also more traditional fields such as "integration of image processing in web-based visualizations" were indicated (participant **I**).

Q10: Where do you see the main obstacles of bringing BioMedVis research results to practice?

Several interviewees see as the main obstacle the collaboration between academia, healthcare, and industry: "There needs to be a deep understanding between these three sectors [...] A major obstacle today is the difficulties for academia and industry to get access to relevant healthcare data. And healthcare needs to boost their capacity to lead innovation and change, especially based on data-driven methods" (participant **L**). Participant **D** remarked that "connecting the developers with the users—not after the fact, but during the development itself" is necessary. However, another participant mentions that "[we need to] connect the two, so that scientific research is potentially relevant for application, without being the servant of it. Co-development is a solution in some cases, but not always" (participant **K**). Several participants see as a big hurdle the necessity for certification and licensing (participants **A**, **E**, **H**), while two more mentioned the "long road from research prototype to actual application" (participants **H** and **E**, who also highlighted that "the lesson learned must go beyond the specific use case").

Participants **P** and **E** discuss another important problem: "It is hard for researchers to build a tool that is at first stable enough for an everyday application and secondly, is not yet another tool in an increasingly complex workflow." "Ph.D. research often solves the first 80% of the problem which have scientific merit (i.e., are publishable), but in practice, the remaining 20% (which are 80% of the work) are not scientifically relevant and not publishable. So they often do not get done." To this last comment, participant **P** added: "the focus of today's research setup on Ph.D. theses and single projects means that increasingly large research teams are favored who build extensive toolkits, [and] only with this basis a Ph.D. student can make a contribution that has a chance in practice." Participant **G** structured the obstacles into being a matter of wrong time, wrong context, wrong individuals, nice-to-have vs. must-have solutions, and research disconnected from what the application needs.

Q11: What are common threats to the future of the field of BioMedVis?

Eight threats were identified, and most of the participants (partially) agree with each other. These are the following. A lack of funding was identified by three people. Two people identified a lack of infrastructure—participant **G** spots a "lack of infrastructure in terms of larger teams" and participant **B** recognizes that "things need to be developed over and over again because we don't have a lot of infrastructure to build upon." Fragmentation of the field was identified by five people. Two people identified wrong goals—participant **G** stated that "BioMedVis, as Vis in general, should carefully identify their special opportunities and avoid competing on grounds where it has lost up-front, e.g., against machine learning" and participant **K** mentions that a problem here is also "blind reliance on AI techniques."

Participant **F** remarked on the loss of young researchers to large companies which academia cannot compete with, while participant **K** additionally commented that "we could also turn this around by aiming for increased collaboration with industry (large or small scale). But also this is not an easy thing to achieve." Further, regarding achieving the right level of complexity, participant **L** stated that "simplicity is an absolute must, and difficult to achieve, but may be seen as a weaker scientific contribution," while participant **E** discussed that "We should try to avoid complicated [but] not really working case studies with no impact." Being able to work with personal, real data in the medical domain was also discussed: "[...] the obstacles that one has to overcome to be able to work with such data are increasing significantly [despite the need for privacy protection]" (participant **P**). Finally, participant **O** mentioned the "possibility that [the fields] are open to abuse."

4.2 Reflective Summary

The interviews have explored various aspects of BioMedVis. Participants have reflected on the "golden age" of BioMedVis, identifying different timeframes and noting ongoing advancements. They discussed solved problems and emerging trends like integrating visualization with machine learning and remarked that even seemingly solved topics such as volume visualization are benefitting from new machine learning methods. Changes in BioMedVis over the years include shifts in research topics, increased data complexity, and advancements in technology. Participants also debated the relationship between BioVis and MedVis, with varying opinions: some consider them tightly related and others totally separate fields. Yet, they unanimously agreed on the importance of BioMedVis due to its potential impact on healthcare and understanding biological systems. Significant past achievements mentioned include volume rendering and visualization of blood flow. Current trends revolve around machine learning integration, data complexity handling, and explainable AI. Open challenges include bridging scales, implementing visualizations effectively, and bringing research results into practice. Future application domains include genomics, population biology, and personalized medicine. Common threats to the field's future include fragmentation, lack of funding, and the risk of losing researchers to industry. Overall, the responses provide insights into the past, present, and potential future of BioMedVis, highlighting its significance and ongoing challenges in advancing healthcare and biological understanding.

5 Discussion

In 2014, Botha et al. [70] published a position paper with a 30-year overview of key developments in the area of medical visualization and their observations on future challenges. They highlighted volume and illustrative visualization, as well as multimodal, multi-field, time-varying, and multi-subject visualization as the main advancements of the field. They foresaw several challenges coming from new data acquisitions and the use of heterogeneous displays and devices, as well as the integration of interactive segmentation, topological approaches, and simulation models. They also emphasized the need for new mappings and reformations, and illustrative vs. hyper-realistic solutions. Visual analytics in healthcare and population imaging have also been among their “predictions.”

Fast-forwarding to today, these predictions were indeed accurate and most are still not fully solved—especially those related to the continuous evolution of data acquisition methods. A recent viewpoint work by Gillmann et al. [192] re-iterates the open challenges in medical visualization. Data preparation, access, and standardization are timely data-specific challenges, while uncertainty, multimodal and multiscale visualization, and evaluation are (or remain) cornerstones. We can find similar challenges also in biology: the recent work of O’Donoghue [448] gives concrete examples of the visualization challenges in bioinformatics dealing with multiscale and multimodal data. Additionally, both viewpoints emphasize the user and the need for communication, with emerging explainable AI, immersive and narrative visualization, and in medicine also personalized, predictive, preventive, and participatory solutions.

In this chapter, we include a confirmation of the evolution of the past topics in the BioMedVis domain obtained through topic modeling. Subsequently, on top of the challenges discussed by Botha et al., Gillmann et al., and O’Donoghue we hereby provide a discussion on subjects that we anticipate to be concerned with in the upcoming years.

K. Furmanová et al., *BioMedical Visualization*, Synthesis Lectures on Visualization,
https://doi.org/10.1007/978-3-031-66789-3_5

5.1 Topic Evolution Modeling

To unbiasedly confirm the *evolution of topics* in the joint domain of MedVis and BioVis, as presented in Chap. 3, we additionally resort to natural language processing (NLP) that helps us to explore the vast number of papers at hand. Our mixed-initiative approach is anticipated to provide a significant addition to the manual categorization shown in Chap. 3, by providing a meaningful suggestion of topics present in the corpus of papers. To obtain this additional dimension, we extracted the abstract and the title from all collected papers. Then, these texts underwent preprocessing: *tokenization* splits the text into sentences and the sentences into words, while all words are lower-cased and punctuation is removed. *Stopwords* (e.g., "*novel*", "*good*", "*user*", etc.) are removed. Then, words are *lemmatized* (i.e., inflected forms of a word are grouped and analyzed together) and *stemmed* (i.e., inflected forms of a word are reduced to their stem).

Subsequently, we applied a Latent Dirichlet Allocation (LDA) approach [59] for topic modeling. LDA is an automatic method for understanding, organizing, and summarizing large electronic archives that can help with discovering topics in a large collection of documents and classifying them into the identified topics. In essence, we use a generative model to classify text from the abstracts and titles to a particular topic modeled as Dirichlet distribution. LDA requires adequate parametrization, for which we conducted a two-step hyper-parameter grid search. After optimal parametrization (learning offset $\tau_0 = 20$ and learning decay $\kappa = 0.9$), LDA yielded 15 topics, which are summarized in Fig. 5.1, together with their most prominent 8 terms.

However, some post-processing was required too. Topic 5 includes keywords such as "*game*", "*microscopy*", "*games*", "*optical*", which do not indicate a coherent topic. This group comprises only 16 papers and, after a closer look, we identified that it mostly included microscopy visualization applications and serious games for biology. We decided to post-process this topic and re-assign the papers to the other topics (8 papers were re-assigned to Topic 9, and 8 papers to Topic 12). Figure 5.2 summarizes the outcomes of the post-processed topic modeling and the assignment of papers to those. The final topics list, ordered by size, is the following:

- Augmented and virtual reality for education, rehabilitation, or surgical applications (740 papers, 19.2% of corpus; Topic 12)
- Volume rendering of medical image data (431 papers, 11.2% of corpus; Topic 2)
- Visualizing biology at different scales: proteins, molecules, and cells (431 papers, 11.2% of corpus; Topic 9)
- Visualizations to support segmentation and registration (345 papers, 8.9% of corpus; Topic 10)
- Visualizing gene expression and genomic sequences (311 papers, 8.1% of corpus; Topic 4)
- Surface rendering for molecular structures (299 papers, 7.8% of corpus; Topic 1)
- Visualizing brain connectivity (205 papers, 5.3% of corpus; Topic 11)

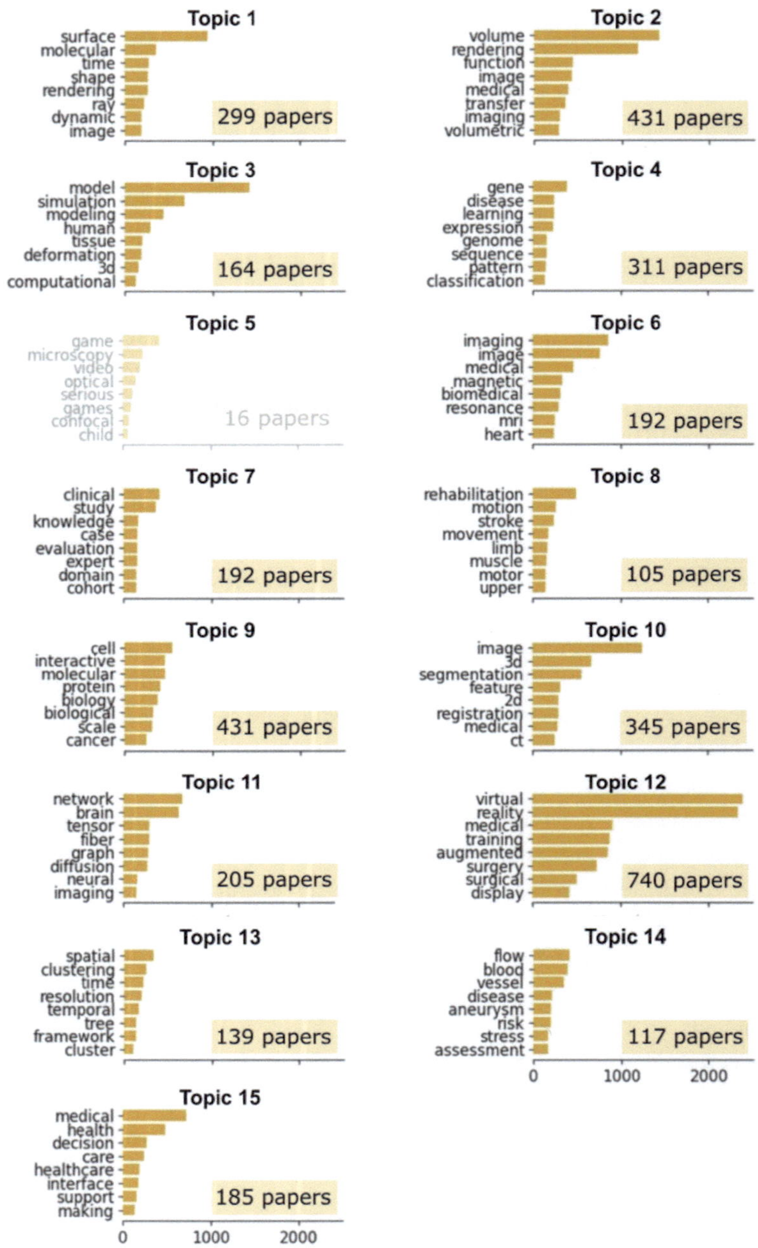

Fig. 5.1 Results of a Latent Dirichlet Allocation (LDA) for topic modeling applied on the corpus of our papers. The LDA (parameter setup for learning offset $\tau_0 = 20$ and for learning decay $\kappa = 0.9$) yielded 15 topics, which are depicted here with their most prominent 8 terms. Bars indicate term frequencies. Topic 5 has been faded out, being an incoherent topic with only 16 papers, which were re-assigned to Topics 9 and 12

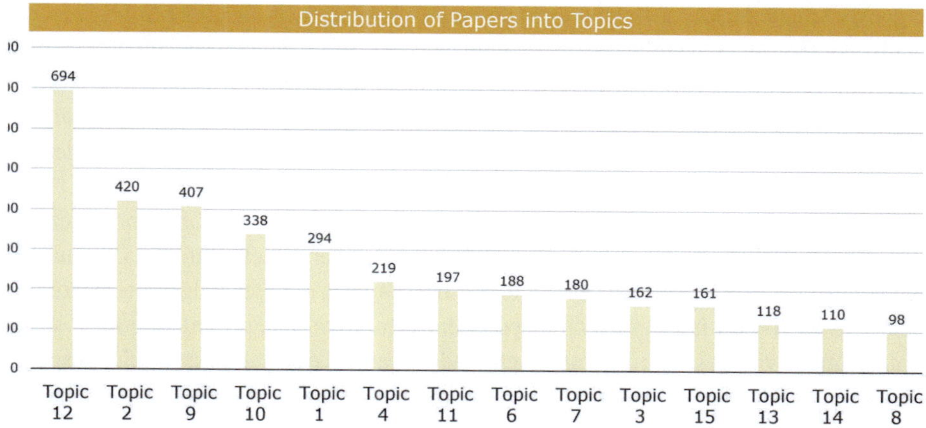

Fig. 5.2 Distribution of the papers in our corpus across topics in decreasing order, as resulting from the post-processed LDA depicted in Fig. 5.1. Note that Topic 5 has been merged with Topics 9 and 12

- Visualizing cardiac data on the basis of MRI medical images (192 papers, 5% of corpus; Topic 6)
- Studies: cohort studies and evaluations (192 papers, 5% of corpus; Topic 7)
- Visualizations for decision-making support (185 papers, 4.8% of corpus; Topic 15)
- Visualizing simulations of human models and tissue deformations (164 papers, 4.3% of corpus; Topic 3)
- Visual analytics for spatial and temporal data (139 papers, 3.6% of corpus; Topic 13)
- Visualizing blood flow and vasculature (117 papers, 3% of corpus; Topic 14)
- Visualizing motion data for rehabilitation (105 papers, 2.7% of corpus; Topic 8).

5.2 Evaluation

With more and more techniques available to visualize biomedical data, the question of which technique is appropriate for which purpose becomes increasingly important. The appropriateness includes technical aspects, such as rendering times and accuracy that may be analyzed in a *validation* [479]. In this section, however, we focus on evaluation which means that *users* are involved to test and assess visualizations among others to measure usability, user experience, and *technology acceptance*.

The appropriateness of visualization techniques depends on the specific data and the target audience. As an example, a vessel visualization technique may be employed for diagnosis with radiologists as the target user group, or for treatment planning with surgeons as the target group, or for science communication with an anticipated broad audience. For diagnosis, small details can be important and thus, visualizations should faithfully represent details. For treatment planning, the branching pattern is often the most essential property of a vascular tree. For a broad audience, even the branching pattern may need to be shown in a simplified manner. Before designing an evaluation study, a careful requirement analysis is necessary and the evaluation should be focused on the question of how well the identified (and verified) requirements are met.

One type of evaluation in biomedical visualization measures a visualization technique with respect to 3D perception, i.e., depth and shape perception. A set of stimuli, i.e., images or video sequences, is created and users accomplish tasks, such as depth judgment (determining which of two stimuli is in front) or shape orientation tasks (determining the local surface normal, often with a gauge figure). Such studies can be easily assessed with respect to accuracy and task completion times. Typically, a new method is compared against a baseline method or against other more advanced methods. This type of study is often encountered in the literature, e.g., [352, 519, 527]. A summary of such evaluations was provided by Preim et al. [483].

Other criteria may be even more important from a practical point-of-view. For clinical applications, it is essential that a visualization technique is appropriate for the problem and trustworthy. For science communication visualization techniques should be *engaging* and *memorable*. While the InfoVis community developed a broad set of evaluation criteria and evaluation strategies [258, 343], in biomedical visualization these criteria are rarely considered. A critical analysis of the evaluation practice in medical visualization with a call to broader and more realistic evaluations was provided by Preim et al. [489]. In particular, one aspect of a realistic evaluation is often not considered. Evaluations are carried out once for a short period of time in a lab, whereas a realistic understanding requires a long-term evaluation that captures also how the use of a system changes over time [577]. Users of visualization techniques and related systems frequently may benefit from techniques that are initially difficult to learn but are quite effective in the long run. Many interactive visualization strategies in radiological workstations demonstrate this.

Our experience has shown that indications of a successful approach include the *early involvement* of the domain experts in the design and their *tight integration* in all iterations of the development, the *adoption rates* after some years, and also passing the "*test-of-time*." Based on these criteria, two very notable MedVis examples are the CPR technique by Kanitsar et al. [287, 288] and also the LifeLines by Plaisant et al. [477]. From the BioVis domain, the most prominent examples are the enhancements (ambient occlusion and contours) for real-time molecular rendering by Tarini et al. [611] and the seminal work of Connolly on the visualization of smooth molecular surfaces [115]. We discuss more notable examples in conjunction with translation to practice, in the upcoming section.

5.3 Translation to (Clinical) Practice

MedVis research is inspired and driven primarily by diagnostic and therapeutic processes and thus, at least partially, by clinical needs. These also impose strict requirements for the robustness and usability of developed solutions. In the BioVis domain, the target scope is narrower, the intended users are typically domain researchers, and the requirements are often less constraining. Yet, in both domains the adoption of visualization research into practice is slow.

We highlight some impressive success stories of visualization research being actually translated into practice. In MedVis, fundamental research on virtual colonoscopy [246] aiming at powerful and high-quality rendering along with efficient navigation was extended towards stable and easy-to-use prototypes. These prototypes were subject to extensive testing and finally evolved into FDA-approved medical products the use of which gets reimbursed. Another success story relates to curved planar reformations (CPR) [287, 288], as discussed in Section 5.2. Different CPR variants and extensions for branching vessels are widespread in radiological workstations and support the diagnosis of cardiovascular diseases. The methods were already developed together with industrial partners and thus focused on the constraints of clinical routine. A further example for the successful transfer to clinical practice is high-quality photorealistic volume rendering. Considerable research in this area was carried out by researchers at the intersection of academic and industry research, such as ENGEL and LJUNG. This research along with some concepts from Kroes et al. [323] lead to the development of *cinematic rendering* [128, 149]. This powerful concept is widely used for advanced diagnosis and medical education.

However, compared to the large amount and variety of medical visualization research, most research results have not been translated into clinical practice. There are various reasons why the research transition stopped at the stage of early prototypes and related publications. Sometimes, there is just *no clear clinical need*. This could explain, for example, why illustrative medical visualization techniques are not used in practice. As also noted in Chap. 4, research is nowadays focusing more and more on applications rather than algorithms, where quite advanced and hardly standardized types of input data are employed. In these situations, *niche applications and complex workflows* are suitable for medical research but are not simple and robust enough for clinical practice. Examples include research on perfusion data, on measured blood flow data, and also research based on biomedical simulation results, such as biomechanics [134] and blood flow simulation [177]. Additionally, most developments where translation was actually successful were started already as *cooperative efforts with industry*. Without the industry focus on a sufficient market and solutions with a manageable complexity, research results are rarely clinically relevant.

In BioVis, the adoption of visualization research is less constrained, and numerous fundamental visualization techniques are commonly used by biology researchers. An example are molecular surfaces [360] or network representations for biomolecular interaction networks [568]. However, similarly to MedVis, many specialized applications never reach a broader audience. A common challenge brought up in Chap. 4 that hampers translation to practice in both domains is the *lack of reusable and sustainable software platforms*. This leads to a lot of time spent on software re-development, which limits the chances of getting beyond the prototype stage. The software is often abandoned when the associated research project ends as there are no resources for its further development and maintenance. At the same time, significant effort has already been put into the development of toolkits such as MITK, VTK, and frameworks such as MEVISLAB or InViwo in MedVis, and MegaMol in BioVis. While these tools are well established and to a certain extent used in the community, they do not fully eliminate the re-implementation problem [504]. This is in part due to the entry barrier of understanding and extending the existing software, partly due to a lack of support and documentation, and partly due to constantly evolving technologies. For example, we are currently experiencing a shift to predominantly web-based solutions that require new technologies and the re-implementation of many existing techniques. On the other hand, web-based solutions are more readily available to researchers, practitioners, and the general public, which can contribute to their adoption into practice. Another trend contributing to the adoption of visualization techniques in BioVis consists of dedicated **`R`** and **`Python`** packages. Even though these often lack the interactivity of fully developed visual analytics applications, they are easier to integrate into existing analytical workflows. This is especially true for visualization packages that can be used in computational notebook interfaces such as JupyterLab.

5.4 Bridging Data from Multiple Scales

Bridging data across multiple scales was brought up in Chap. 4 as a main challenge that BioMedVis is currently facing. This was already a significant topic in the position paper of Botha et al. [70]. We can identify several reasons why this remains a challenge even though many of the visualization problems at individual scales are solved—at least partially.

Visualization research is to a large extent *task-driven* and develops according to the needs of its *target users*. While visualizing the full body of a person with all available data from organ level to atomic level seems like an exciting scientific prospect, biology, and medicine are comprised of a myriad of sub-fields often focusing only on a very narrow spectrum of scales. The need to span many or all scales is not fully there yet, though undoubtedly, bridging the scales and providing a bigger picture would be beneficial for many areas of biomedicine. For example, there are currently efforts to associate omics with medicine, e.g., in the context of personalized treatment or for biomarker identification. Such efforts, though, should start with a definition of objectives. For instance, BioVis has often focused on exploratory analysis, while MedVis has had a more explanatory nature. This naturally also requires a collaboration between experts from sub-fields of biomedicine.

Another reason for not going across many scales is the *lack of information* between the available resolutions. To some extent, this is continuously improved by technological advancements for data acquisition as well as computational modeling that could fill in the gaps. However, in some areas, we are still facing the problem of missing data links (common parameters and attributes) that make it difficult to relate datasets from different scales. It still remains a challenge to, for example, connect radiology with proteomics or genomics—also due to practical reasons (e.g., resolution or registration). In other areas opportunities supporting bridging the scales can be found. For example, Garrison et al. [175] have discussed the opportunities for multiscale visualization in physiology.

Another problem is the *complexity* of the data—beyond the computational power required for the handling of multiscale datasets. The challenge relates also to data heterogeneity occurring in biomedicine; including spatial, abstract, multi-dimensional, or temporal data. Designing visual mappings to combine multiple datatypes is not trivial and might lead to issues with available visual channels, e.g., limited use of colors and their re-use at different scales. Transitioning between scales has been researched to some extent for spatial data, e.g., in molecular visualization [409]. However, the combination of heterogeneous data from vastly different scales remains largely unexplored. Besides the visual mapping problem, the complexity of such data also presents a cognitive challenge for the user. In this respect, guidance, navigation, and storytelling principles can be helpful.

5.5 Bridging BioVis and MedVis

As we discussed throughout this book, biology and medicine are tightly connected fields by nature and cannot exist without each other. Therefore, it is reasonable to assume that these two areas, as well as their related fields (e.g., visualization), share many similarities. In the visualization domain, there have already been numerous discussions about the overlap of biology and medicine in tasks and requirements that can be supported by similar visual representations. Such discussions also led to the initiation of the Eurographics workshop series on Visual Computing in Biology and Medicine in 2007, or to a number of Dagstuhl and Shonan seminars.

The visual support intrinsically follows the individual methods that we encounter in the two fields and we evidence methods that are present in one of the fields and missing in the other one. An example is segmentation—one of the most basic tasks in medicine that has little presence in the biological domain, where the data are often abstract or modeled rather than image-based. Oppositely, many techniques are employed in both fields. Volume rendering is a basic method in medical visualization and finds its place also in biology—for example to study the occupancy of the molecular volume by its atoms over time. Another example is the study of large data ensembles, where information visualization techniques combined into visual analysis tools are successfully applied. In medicine, an example are cohort studies of large multi-dimensional patient data. In biology, we can explore large datasets of molecules with their diverse properties as potential candidates for new drugs.

Although we recognize these overlaps on the level of individual examples, we are still missing a conceptualization of the relationship between biological and medical visualization. With an increased focus on applied solutions, the convergence of research directions between BioVis and MedVis is challenging to a greater extent. This results in a limited shared knowledge between the domains and also a limited transfer of techniques from one field to the other. To overcome this, we can start by educating visualization students interested in biology or medicine and devise a shared curriculum that targets the commonalities between biological and medical visualizations.

Additionally, several applications lend themselves and actually demand a close cross-domain collaboration. As discussed in the previous section, this is natural in bridging scales (e.g., for —omics in personalized medicine) and in dealing with the mesoscale and the gap that it currently exhibits. Both fields often discuss science communication to general audiences and the democratization of knowledge to the public. Therefore, the domains of BioVis and MedVis may find opportunities to work closer together—especially, in conjunction with research topics such as narrative visualization or physicalization.

5.6 Opportunities for Best Practices

Data Protection. The rules for the protection of biomedical data are (and should be) strict—falling under the personal data provisions of the GDPR. This has been a recurrent topic, even before the recent legislation [70]. Anonymizing biomedical data is challenging: even if a CT scan only has an anonymous ID assigned to it, the data are rather pseudo-anonymous. With high-resolution scans, the identity of a patient might also be retrievable (e.g., through a rendering of a head CT scan). Thus, the creation of a repository of real and synthetic datasets would be useful for testing new visualization techniques or strategies with fewer ethical/privacy implications—even for benchmarking purposes.

Data Integration and Standardization. The ongoing biomedical data explosion comes also at a cost of data quality in terms of integration (i.e., all available information is consistently integrated to enable joint analysis) and standardization (i.e., all available information is comparable). Both aspects should be ensured. A fruitful direction towards this requires the curation of a benchmark repository that guarantees inclusiveness by interchange formats and by logging metadata to record provenance [192]. This will allow us to associate data with publications for reproducibility and calibration reasons (similar to Nature Scientific Data practices).

Homo Universalis. A common agreement is that working in the BioMedVis domain requires obtaining early and profound knowledge of the respective life sciences or medical domains. Additionally, various technical expertises are required, e.g., visualization, image processing, image analysis, and machine learning. We see clear advantages of collocating BioMedVis events with other meetings, which could be either from an application or an adjacent technical domain. Further, we should support with our participation venues of local domains of expertise, e.g., local medical or bioinformatics conferences. These are excellent sources for new ideas and new collaborations.

Adoptability and Conventions. The focus of BioMedVis research needs to provide visualization solutions for the medical or biological domain. It has to consider both the employed technical methodologies and the addressed application domain. We often face the problem of ensuring adoptability. A main obstacle in this is the contradicting nature of conventions in the domain and the adequacy (or even correctness) of the visualization design. A common example is the use of rainbow color maps. Despite its many perceptual flaws, it remains the most common color map in clinical practice. Putting extra effort into obtaining deeper knowledge about the application domain and meaningful conventions is of utmost importance. This increases the chances to develop useful solutions with features that are must-haves, rather than nice-to-haves. An "easy" way to achieve this is for visualization experts to work for some time directly in the environment of the domain experts. This allows them to co-design strategies to tackle domain problems, organize semi-structured workshops with domain experts (preferably from different institutions), and team up with companies to make sure that the visual design is not compromised.

Reusability and Sustainability. There is currently a large collection of prototypes, visual designs, techniques, and development kits, which are hard to generalize and extend to other domains. Healthy ecosystems, such as **R** in the statistics community, make it possible to require a compatible implementation alongside a publication. Yet, in our community, there is a perceived lack of incentives for the extra effort to create and maintain reusable visualization software. An increased focus on larger collaborative community projects would lead to a much more efficient use of resources. Having a curated list of visualization software and repositories, as well as the use of reproducibility and sustainability badges are good additional incentives.

On Artificial Intelligence (AI). The best practices in AI for BioMedVis comprise a convergence of cutting-edge technology, ethical considerations, and collaborative efforts aimed at advancing healthcare and research. To begin, the sensitive nature of medical information necessitates robust measures to protect it from unauthorized access or breaches. Moreover, transparency in AI algorithms and models is fundamental. Providing clinicians, researchers, and end-users with a clear understanding of how AI systems operate and arrive at their conclusions enhances trust and confidence, and encourages adoption—for instance, by making use of new explainable AI concepts among which is also guidance. By pooling collective expertise, domain experts, data scientists, and healthcare professionals can tailor AI solutions to address specific biomedical challenges and optimize patient care. Regular validation and rigorous testing of AI systems are essential to maintain accuracy and reliability. The dynamic nature of medical knowledge requires continuous updates and refinements to AI models to ensure they remain current and effective. With the advent of generative AI, there are new opportunities to revolutionize biomedical visualization by creating synthetic data for training, enhancing imaging resolution, and facilitating data augmentation. It can also streamline complex analyses and enable personalized visualizations, advancing both research and clinical applications—also in terms of usability, for instance through onboarding. On the other side, Large Language Models can transform biomedical visualization by assisting in data interpretation, generating descriptive labels, and providing context for visualizations. In all these cases, AI in biomedical visualization must operate within the boundaries of established legal and ethical frameworks, taking into account factors like informed consent, bias mitigation, and accountability.

Certification. Quality assurance is another challenge in BioMedVis when transferring research software into clinical practice (see also Sect. 5.3). Strong certification regulations (e.g., FDA) are in place for all software that influences patient care decisions—going beyond the trust of a clinician. Often, prototypes, e.g., developed by an (under)graduate student, are way below the high standards required for certification, and it would be unreasonable to demand otherwise. A close collaboration with industrial partners can prove beneficial if they are familiar with and willing to undergo the strenuous certification processes.

Accessibility. Accessibility is the practice of making software (and research outcomes, in general) available to as many people within the intended target group as possible. In visualization, we often discuss accessibility in terms of open-source development, web-based applications, and strategies for mobile devices or devices with limited throughput and resolution. Additionally, there is a discourse about open research. We do not often talk about making software accessible to disabilities—with the exception of color deficiencies. Semantic accessibility is one of the main flavors of accessibility that targets specifically people with visual, hearing, and mobility impairments. It makes use of assistive technologies such as screen readers, captions and transcripts, and keyboard accessibility or other types of pointers, respectively. Still, solutions for cognitive impairment need to be better formalized, e.g., guidance focusing attention on important content or use of familiar elements. Considering accessibility implications from the beginning of the project should be standard practice—especially in web-based applications or when targeting general audiences. This brings new challenges in development, implementation, and evaluation.

Outreach and Dissemination. Visualization research is usually published in specialized journals that, due to the community size, have a rather low impact factor compared to other disciplines. To increase the visibility of our work, we recommend putting extra effort into showcasing results, methods, and tools beyond the visualization community. This can include social media outreach, making source code available, creating demos and tutorials, or promoting the work in application domain venues and exhibitions.

Science Communication. BioMedVis yields an unprecedented benefit for science communication by providing a natural means for informing, educating, or raising awareness about healthcare topics. As more and more approaches address patients and the general audiences, BioMedVis can use storytelling, narrative approaches, metaphors, illustrations, infographics, etc. to communicate (new) scientific concepts in ways explicitly designed to address the literacy, age, and expertise of the audience. This can be of particular benefit to domains such as public health and epidemiology policy making, but also for the engaging education of the masses about anatomy, biology, and common pathologies. Patient communication is a special case, where the patients are informed in a clear manner about their conditions by their doctors. They can also be subsequently involved in making treatment decisions. In BioMedVis research there is currently a lack of evidence-based science communication to bridge research and practice. This presents new opportunities for the future, especially with regard to the educational benefits of visualization.

6 Conclusion

In this book, we provided an overview of trends in biological and medical visualization from the early beginnings until now. To trace the evolution of the trends over the years, we conducted extensive literature research that yielded more than 3,800 publications. We manually categorized the results according to a five-dimensional taxonomy and provided an overview of the topics within the explored literature. An online, interactive repository with our publication collection was made available to the community for further use at https://biomedvis-book.fi.muni.cz/. We further analyzed and discussed literature with respect to temporal developments and changes in research focus within individual application areas. To get a broader perspective on the entire field we also conducted interviews with 16 BioMedVis researchers, collecting their opinions on the evolution of the field.

What are the overall trends through the years? How are the topics evolving with the course of time? Where is the field heading in the upcoming decade? These were the three questions, that we posed at the beginning of the book. We now take a look back and, generalizing our findings, we make the following observations.

Overall, we see a shift from visualizations focused on data representation (e.g., volume rendering) to highly interactive approaches supporting complex analysis and exploration of patterns and relationships. This observation is supported by the declining number of publications focused on general representation techniques that we discussed in Chap. 2 and it can also be seen in the evolution of topics discussed in Chap. 3. For example, in molecular visualization, the focus has largely shifted from the visualization of molecular structures to the analysis of complex simulation datasets. Similarly, in the medical domain, we often see a shift from data of an individual to large cohort studies.

Additionally, major changes in research priorities often result from the development of breakthrough technologies. Notable examples are new imaging techniques, GPU rendering, AR/VR technologies, web-browsing technologies, artificial intelligence, and large language

K. Furmanová et al., *BioMedical Visualization*, Synthesis Lectures on Visualization,
https://doi.org/10.1007/978-3-031-66789-3_6

models. These aspects are also related to a constant increase in data size and complexity, affecting the evolution of the field. However, not all areas are equally affected by the changes. For example, the size of molecular dynamic simulations has increased at least by three orders of magnitude over the years, driving the need for different data analysis approaches. On the other hand, in radiological imaging, the growth of the data size is much slower—although multimodal, multiscale, or cohort-based approaches are nowadays prominent.

In the coming years, new methods of data acquisition might prompt the development of novel data representation techniques. Existing techniques might also benefit from further technological advances, as is currently the case with AI (e.g., generative models and Large Language Models). A notable example of this is the Neural Radiance Field (NeRF) application for medical imaging. We envision that the trend of shifting "from the lower hanging fruits to more complex, larger datasets and application areas," as expressed by one of the interviewed researchers in Chap. 4, will continue. In Chap. 5 we further discussed several topics that we expect to become increasingly important in the upcoming years with regard to evaluation, bridging data from multiple scales and between Bio- and MedVis, translating developments to clinical practices, and best practices in the field. We eagerly anticipate the wealth of insights biomedical visualization can further offer, empowering researchers to unravel the complexities of datasets and articulate intricate biological phenomena with greater clarity and effectiveness.

References

1. Abbasloo, A., Wiens, V., Hermann, M., Schultz, T.: Visualizing tensor normal distributions at multiple levels of detail. IEEE Trans. Vis. Comput. Graph. **22**(1), 975–984 (2015). https://doi.org/10.1109/TVCG.2015.2467031
2. Achenbach, S., Moshage, W., Ropers, D., Bachmann, K.: Curved multiplanar reconstructions for the evaluation of contrast-enhanced electron beam CT of the coronary arteries. Am. J. Roentgenol. **170**(4), 895–899 (1998). https://doi.org/10.2214/ajr.170.4.9530029
3. Adams, R., Finn, P., Moes, E., Flannery, K., Rizzo, A.S.: Distractibility in attention/deficit/hyperactivity disorder (ADHD): the virtual reality classroom. Child Neuropsychol. **15**(2), 120–135 (2009). https://doi.org/10.1080/09297040802169077
4. Adams, R., Stancampiano, B., McKenna, M., Small, D.: Case study: a virtual environment for genomic data visualization. In: Proceeding of IEEE Visualization, pp. 513–516 (2002). https://doi.org/10.1109/VISUAL.2002.1183818
5. Afzal, S., Ghani, S., Jenkins-Smith, H.C., Ebert, D.S., Hadwiger, M., Hoteit, I.: A visual analytics based decision making environment for COVID-19 modeling and visualization. In: Proceeding of IEEE Visualization, pp. 86–90 (2020). https://doi.org/10.1109/vis47514.2020.00024
6. Afzal, S., Maciejewski, R., Ebert, D.S.: Visual analytics decision support environment for epidemic modeling and response evaluation. In: Proceeding of IEEE Symposium on Visual Analytics Science and Technology, pp. 191–200 (2011). https://doi.org/10.1109/vast.2011.6102457
7. Agus, M., Calì, C., Al-Awami, A., Gobbetti, E., Magistretti, P., Hadwiger, M.: Interactive volumetric visual analysis of glycogen-derived energy absorption in nanometric brain structures. Comput. Graph. Forum **38**(3), 427–439 (2019). https://doi.org/10.1111/CGF.13700
8. Aigner, W., Miksch, S.: CareVis: integrated visualization of computerized protocols and temporal patient data. Artif. Intell. Med. **37**(3), 203–218 (2006). https://doi.org/10.1016/j.artmed.2006.04.002
9. Akkiraju, N., Edelsbrunner, H., Fu, P., Qian, J.: Viewing geometric protein structures from inside a CAVE. IEEE Comput. Graph. Appl. **16**(4), 58–61 (1996). https://doi.org/10.1109/38.511855
10. Al-Awami, A.K., Beyer, J., Strobelt, H., Kasthuri, N., Lichtman, J.W., Pfister, H., Hadwiger, M.: Neurolines: a subway map metaphor for visualizing nanoscale neuronal connectivity.

K. Furmanová et al., *BioMedical Visualization*, Synthesis Lectures on Visualization,
https://doi.org/10.1007/978-3-031-66789-3

IEEE Trans. Vis. Comput. Graph. **20**(12), 2369–2378 (2014). https://doi.org/10.1109/tvcg.2014.2346312

11. Al-Hiyari, N., Jusoh, S.: The current trends of virtual reality applications in medical education. In: Proceeding of Electronics, Computers and Artificial Intelligence, pp. 1–6 (2020). https://doi.org/10.1109/ECAI50035.2020.9223158
12. Al-Thelaya, K., Agus, M., Gilal, N.U., Yang, Y., Pintore, G., Gobbetti, E., Calí, C., Magistretti, P.J., Mifsud, W., Schneider, J.: InShaDe: invariant shape descriptors for visual 2D and 3D cellular and nuclear shape analysis and classification. Comput. Graph. **98**, 105–125 (2021). https://doi.org/10.1016/j.cag.2021.04.037
13. Albers, D., Dewey, C., Gleicher, M.: Sequence surveyor: leveraging overview for scalable genomic alignment visualization. IEEE Trans. Vis. Comput. Graph. **17**(12), 2392–2401 (2011). https://doi.org/10.1109/tvcg.2011.232
14. Alemzadeh, S., Hielscher, T., Niemann, U., Cibulski, L., Ittermann, T., Völzke, H., Spiliopoulou, M., Preim, B.: Subpopulation discovery and validation in epidemiological data. In: Proceeding of EuroVis Workshop on Visual Analytics, pp. 43–47 (2017). https://doi.org/10.2312/eurova.20171118
15. Alemzadeh, S., Niemann, U., Ittermann, T., Völzke, H., Schneider, D., Spiliopoulou, M., Bühler, K., Preim, B.: Visual analysis of missing values in longitudinal cohort study data. Comput. Graph. Forum **39**(1), 63–75 (2020). https://doi.org/10.1111/cgf.13662
16. Alharbi, N., Alharbi, M., Martinez, X., Krone, M., Rose, A.S., Baaden, M., Laramee, R.S., Chavent, M.: Molecular visualization of computational biology data: a survey of surveys. In: Proceeding of EuroVis—Short Papers (2017). https://doi.org/10.2312/eurovisshort.20171146
17. Alharbi, N., Krone, M., Chavent, M., Laramee, R.S.: Hybrid visualization of protein-lipid and protein-protein interaction. In: Proceeding of Eurographics Workshop on Visual Computing for Biology and Medicine, pp. 213–223 (2019). https://doi.org/10.2312/VCBM.20191247
18. Amir, E.a.D., Davis, K.L., Tadmor, M.D., Simonds, E.F., Levine, J.H., Bendall, S.C., Shenfeld, D.K., Krishnaswamy, S., Nolan, G.P., Pe'er, D.: viSNE enables visualization of high dimensional single-cell data and reveals phenotypic heterogeneity of leukemia. Nat. Biotechnol. **31**(6), 545–552 (2013). https://doi.org/10.1038/nbt.2594
19. Ang, K.D., Samavati, F.F., Sabokrohiyeh, S., Garcia, J., Elbaz, M.S.: Physicalizing cardiac blood flow data via 3D printing. Comput. Graph. **85**, 42–54 (2019). https://doi.org/10.1016/J.CAG.2019.09.004
20. Angenent, S., Haker, S., Tannenbaum, A., Kikinis, R.: On the Laplace-Beltrami operator and brain surface flattening. IEEE Trans. Med. Imaging **18**(8), 700–711 (1999). https://doi.org/10.1109/42.796283
21. Antiga, L., Piccinelli, M., Botti, L., Ene-Iordache, B., Remuzzi, A., Steinman, D.A.: An image-based modeling framework for patient-specific computational hemodynamics. Med. Biol. Eng. Comput. **46**(11), 1097–1112 (2008). https://doi.org/10.1007/S11517-008-0420-1
22. Arens, S., Domik, G.: A survey of transfer functions suitable for volume rendering. In: Proceeding of IEEE/EG Symposium on Volume Graphics (2010). https://doi.org/10.2312/VG/VG10/077-083
23. Arlati, S., Colombo, V., Ferrigno, G., Sacchetti, R., Sacco, M.: Virtual reality-based wheelchair simulators: a scoping review. Assist. Technol. **32**(6), 294–305 (2020). https://doi.org/10.1080/10400435.2018.1553079
24. Aupetit, M., Ullah, E., Rawi, R., Bensmail, H.: A design study to identify inconsistencies in kinship information: the case of the 1000 Genomes project. In: Proceeding of IEEE Pacific Visualization Symposium (2016). https://doi.org/10.1109/pacificvis.2016.7465281
25. Aurisano, J., Reda, K., Johnson, A., Leigh, J.: Bacterial gene neighborhood investigation environment: a large-scale genome visualization for big displays. In: Proceeding of IEEE Sym-

posium on Large Data Analysis and Visualization (2014). https://doi.org/10.1109/ldav.2014.7013210
26. Ayobi, A., Marshall, P., Cox, A.L.: Trackly: a customisable and pictorial self-tracking app to support agency in multiple sclerosis self-care. In: Proceeding of the CHI Conference on Human Factors in Computing Systems, pp. 1–15 (2020). https://doi.org/10.1145/3313831.3376809
27. Azimi, E., Liu, R., Molina, C., Huang, J., Kazanzides, P.: Interactive navigation system in mixed-reality for neurosurgery. In: Proceeding of IEEE Conference on Virtual Reality and 3D User Interfaces Abstracts and Workshops, pp. 782–783 (2020). https://doi.org/10.1109/vrw50115.2020.00242
28. Bade, R., Haase, J., Preim, B.: Comparison of fundamental mesh smoothing algorithms for medical surface models. In: Proceeding of SimVis, vol. 6, pp. 289–304 (2006)
29. Baer, A., Tietjen, C., Bade, R., Preim, B.: Hardware-accelerated stippling of surfaces derived from medical volume data. In: Proceeding of EuroVis, pp. 235–242 (2007). https://doi.org/10.2312/VISSYM/EUROVIS07/235-242
30. Bai, X.C., McMullan, G., Scheres, S.H.: How cryo-EM is revolutionizing structural biology. Trends Biochem. Sci. **40**(1), 49–57 (2015). https://doi.org/10.1016/j.tibs.2014.10.005
31. Bai, Z., Blackwell, A.F., Coulouris, G.: Using augmented reality to elicit pretend play for children with autism. IEEE Trans. Vis. Comput. Graph. **21**(5), 598–610 (2014). https://doi.org/10.1109/TVCG.2014.2385092
32. Ban, Y.E.A., Edelsbrunner, H., Rudolph, J.: Interface surfaces for protein-protein complexes. J. ACM **53**(3), 361–378 (2006). https://doi.org/10.1145/1147954.1147957
33. Barsky, A., Gardy, J.L., Hancock, R.E.W., Munzner, T.: Cerebral: a Cytoscape plugin for layout of and interaction with biological networks using subcellular localization annotation. Bioinformatics **23**(8), 1040–1042 (2007). https://doi.org/10.1093/bioinformatics/btm057
34. Barsky, A., Munzner, T., Gardy, J., Kincaid, R.: Cerebral: visualizing multiple experimental conditions on a graph with biological context. IEEE Trans. Vis. Comput. Graph. **14**(6), 1253–1260 (2008). https://doi.org/10.1109/tvcg.2008.117
35. Basdogan, C., Sedef, M., Harders, M., Wesarg, S.: VR-based simulators for training in minimally invasive surgery. IEEE Comput. Graph. Appl. **27**(2), 54–66 (2007). https://doi.org/10.1109/mcg.2007.51
36. Battke, F., Symons, S., Nieselt, K.: Mayday-integrative analytics for expression data. BMC Bioinformatics **11**(1), 121 (2010). https://doi.org/10.1186/1471-2105-11-121
37. Bauer, A., Paclet, F., Cahouet, V., Dicko, A.H., Palombi, O., Faure, F., Troccaz, J.: Interactive visualization of muscle activity during limb movements: towards enhanced anatomy learning. In: Proceeding of Eurographics Workshop on Visual Computing for Biology and Medicine, pp. 191–198 (2014). https://doi.org/10.2312/vcbm.20141191
38. Bayrak, R.G., Hoang, N., Hansen, C.B., Chang, C., Berger, M.: PRAGMA: interactively constructing functional brain parcellations. In: Proceeding of IEEE Visualization, pp. 46–50 (2020). https://doi.org/10.1109/vis47514.2020.00016
39. Becher, B., Schlitzer, A., Chen, J., Mair, F., Sumatoh, H.R., Teng, K.W.W., Low, D., Ruedl, C., Riccardi-Castagnoli, P., Poidinger, M., Greter, M., Ginhoux, F., Newell, E.W.: High-dimensional analysis of the murine myeloid cell system. Nat. Immunol. **15**(12), 1181–1189 (2014). https://doi.org/10.1038/ni.3006
40. Becht, E., McInnes, L., Healy, J., Dutertre, C.A., Kwok, I.W.H., Ng, L.G., Ginhoux, F., Newell, E.W.: Dimensionality reduction for visualizing single-cell data using UMAP. Nat. Biotechnol. **37**(1), 38–44 (2018). https://doi.org/10.1038/nbt.4314
41. Bedoucha, P., Reuter, N., Hauser, H., Byška, J.: Visual exploration of large normal mode spaces to study protein flexibility. Comput. Graph. **90**, 73–83 (2020). https://doi.org/10.1016/j.cag.2020.05.025

42. Behrendt, B., Berg, P., Preim, B., Saalfeld, S.: Combining pseudo chroma depth enhancement and parameter mapping for vascular surface models. In: Proceeding of Eurographics Workshop on Visual Computing in Biology and Medicine, pp. 159–168 (2017). https://doi.org/10.2312/VCBM.20171250
43. Behrendt, B., Pleuss-Engelhardt, D., Gutberlet, M., Preim, B.: 2.5 D geometric mapping of aortic blood flow data for cohort visualization. In: Proceeding of Eurographics Workshop on Visual Computing in Biology and Medicine, pp. 91–100 (2021). https://doi.org/10.2312/VCBM.20211348
44. Belkina, A.C., Ciccolella, C.O., Anno, R., Halpert, R., Spidlen, J., Snyder-Cappione, J.E.: Automated optimized parameters for T-distributed stochastic neighbor embedding improve visualization and analysis of large datasets. Nat. Commun. **10**(1) (2019). https://doi.org/10.1038/s41467-019-13055-y
45. Bello, F., Bulpitt, A., Gould, D.A., Holbrey, R., Hunt, C., How, T., John, N.W., Johnson, S., Phillips, R., Sinha, A., et al.: ImaGiNe-S: imaging guided needle simulation. In: Proceeding of Eurographics—Medical Prize, pp. 5–8 (2009). https://doi.org/10.2312/EGM.20091024
46. Benali, A., Richard, P., Bidaud, P.: A six DOF haptic interface for medical virtual reality applications: design, control and human factors. In: Proceeding of IEEE Virtual Reality, p. 284 (2000). https://doi.org/10.1109/vr.2000.840512
47. Bendall, S.C., Davis, K.L., ad David Amir, E., Tadmor, M.D., Simonds, E.F., Chen, T.J., Shenfeld, D.K., Nolan, G.P., Pe'er, D.: Single-cell trajectory detection uncovers progression and regulatory coordination in human B cell development. Cell **157**(3), 714–725 (2014). https://doi.org/10.1016/j.cell.2014.04.005
48. Schulte zu Berge, C., Weiss, J., Navab, N.: Schematic electrode map for navigation in neuro data sets. In: Proceeding of Eurographics Workshop on Visual Computing in Biology and Medicine, pp. 195–204 (2015). https://doi.org/10.2312/VCBM.20151223
49. Bernard, J., Sessler, D., May, T., Schlomm, T., Pehrke, D., Kohlhammer, J.: A visual-interactive system for prostate cancer cohort analysis. IEEE Comput. Graph. Appl. **35**(3), 44–55 (2015). https://doi.org/10.1109/mcg.2015.49
50. Berres, A., Goldau, M., Tittgemeyer, M., Scheuermann, G., Hagen, H.: Tractography in context: multimodal visualization of probabilistic tractograms in anatomical context. In: Proceeding of Eurographics Workshop on Visual Computing in Biology and Medicine, pp. 9–16 (2012). https://doi.org/10.2312/VCBM/VCBM12/009-016
51. Beyer, J., Al-Awami, A., Kasthuri, N., Lichtman, J.W., Pfister, H., Hadwiger, M.: ConnectomeExplorer: query-guided visual analysis of large volumetric neuroscience data. IEEE Trans. Vis. Comput. Graph. **19**(12), 2868–2877 (2013). https://doi.org/10.1109/tvcg.2013.142
52. Beyer, J., Hadwiger, M., Al-Awami, A., Jeong, W.K., Kasthuri, N., Lichtman, J.W., Pfister, H.: Exploring the connectome: petascale volume visualization of microscopy data streams. IEEE Comput. Graph. Appl. **33**(4), 50–61 (2013). https://doi.org/10.1109/mcg.2013.55
53. Beyer, J., Hadwiger, M., Pfister, H.: State-of-the-art in GPU-based large-scale volume visualization. Comput. Graph. Forum **34**(8), 13–37 (2015). https://doi.org/10.1111/CGF.12605
54. Beyer, J., Hadwiger, M., Wolfsberger, S., Bühler, K.: High-quality multimodal volume rendering for preoperative planning of neurosurgical interventions. IEEE Trans. Vis. Comput. Graph. **13**(6), 1696–1703 (2007). https://doi.org/10.1109/tvcg.2007.70560
55. Beyer, J., Troidl, J., Boorboor, S., Hadwiger, M., Kaufman, A., Pfister, H.: A survey of visualization and analysis in high-resolution connectomics. Comput. Graph. Forum **41**(3), 573–607 (2022). https://doi.org/10.1111/CGF.14574
56. Bichlmeier, C., Euler, E., Blum, T., Navab, N.: Evaluation of the virtual mirror as a navigational aid for augmented reality driven minimally invasive procedures. In: Proceeding of IEEE International Symposium on Mixed and Augmented Reality, pp. 91–97 (2010). https://doi.org/10.1109/ismar.2010.5643555

57. Blaas, J., Botha, C.P., Peters, B., Vos, F.M., Post, F.H.: Fast and reproducible fiber bundle selection in DTI visualization. In: Proceeding of IEEE Visualization, pp. 59–64 (2005). https://doi.org/10.1109/VISUAL.2005.1532778
58. Black, D., Hettig, J., Luz, M., Hansen, C., Kikinis, R., Hahn, H.: Auditory feedback to support image-guided medical needle placement. Int. J. Comput. Assist. Radiol. Surg. **12**(9), 1655–1663 (2017). https://doi.org/10.1007/s11548-017-1537-1
59. Blei, D.M., Ng, A.Y., Jordan, M.I.: Latent dirichlet allocation. J. Mach. Learn. Res. **3**, 993–1022 (2003)
60. Bloomenthal, J., Shoemake, K.: Convolution surfaces. In: Proceeding of Computer Graphics and Interactive Techniques, pp. 251–256 (1991). https://doi.org/10.1145/122718.122757
61. Blum, T., Heining, S.M., Kutter, O., Navab, N.: Advanced training methods using an augmented reality ultrasound simulator. In: Proceeding of IEEE International Symposium on Mixed and Augmented Reality, pp. 177–178 (2009). https://doi.org/10.1109/ismar.2009.5336476
62. Blum, T., Kleeberger, V., Bichlmeier, C., Navab, N.: mirracle: An augmented reality magic mirror system for anatomy education. In: Proceeding of IEEE Virtual Reality Workshops, pp. 115–116 (2012). https://doi.org/10.1109/vr.2012.6180909
63. Blume, A., Chun, W., Kogan, D., Kokkevis, V., Weber, N., Petterson, R.W., Zeiger, R.: Google body: 3D human anatomy in the browser. In: Proceeding of ACM SIGGRAPH—Talks, p. 19 (2011). https://doi.org/10.1145/2037826.2037852
64. Bock, A., Lang, N., Evangelista, G., Lehrke, R., Ropinski, T.: Guiding deep brain stimulation interventions by fusing multimodal uncertainty regions. In: Proceeding of IEEE Pacific Visualization Symposium, pp. 97–104 (2013). https://doi.org/10.1109/pacificvis.2013.6596133
65. Boissonnat, J.D., Geiger, B.: 3D simulation of delivery. In: Proceeding of IEEE Visualization, pp. 416–419 (1993). https://doi.org/10.1109/visual.1993.398903
66. Bork, F., Fuers, B., Schneider, A.K., Pinto, F., Graumann, C., Navab, N.: Auditory and visio-temporal distance coding for 3-dimensional perception in medical augmented reality. In: Proceeding of IEEE International Symposium on Mixed and Augmented Reality, pp. 7–12 (2015). https://doi.org/10.1109/ismar.2015.16
67. Born, S., Markl, M., Gutberlet, M., Scheuermann, G.: Illustrative visualization of cardiac and aortic blood flow from 4D MRI data. In: Proceeding of IEEE Pacific Visualization Symposium, pp. 129–136 (2013). https://doi.org/10.1109/pacificvis.2013.6596137
68. Born, S., Pfeifle, M., Markl, M., Gutberlet, M., Scheuermann, G.: Visual analysis of cardiac 4D MRI blood flow using line predicates. IEEE Trans. Vis. Comput. Graph. **19**(6), 900–912 (2012). https://doi.org/10.1109/TVCG.2012.318
69. Born, S., Wiebel, A., Friedrich, J., Scheuermann, G., Bartz, D.: Illustrative stream surfaces. IEEE Trans. Vis. Comput. Graph. **16**(6), 1329–1338 (2010). https://doi.org/10.1109/tvcg.2010.166
70. Botha, C.P., Preim, B., Kaufman, A.E., Takahashi, S., Ynnerman, A.: From individual to population: challenges in medical visualization. In: Scientific Visualization, pp. 265–282. Springer (2014). https://doi.org/10.1007/978-1-4471-6497-523
71. Bourqui, R., Auber, D., Lacroix, V., Jourdan, F.: Metabolic network visualization using constraint planar graph drawing algorithm. In: Proceeding of Information Visualisation, pp. 489–496 (2006).https://doi.org/10.1109/iv.2006.75
72. Bouyer, G., Bourdot, P., Ammi, M.: Supervision of 3D multimodal rendering for protein-protein virtual docking. In: Proceeding of IPT/EGVE, pp. 49–56 (2008). https://doi.org/10.2312/EGVE/EGVE08/049-056
73. Bozorgi, M., Lindseth, F.: GPU-based multi-volume ray casting within VTK for medical applications. Int. J. Comput. Assist. Radiol. Surg. **10**, 293–300 (2014). https://doi.org/10.1007/s11548-014-1069-x

74. Brand, A., Gao, L., Hamann, A., Crayen, C., Brand, H., Squier, S.M., Stangl, K., Kendel, F., Stangl, V.: Medical graphic narratives to improve patient comprehension and periprocedural anxiety before coronary angiography and percutaneous coronary intervention: a randomized trial. Ann. Intern. Med. **170**(8), 579–581 (2019). https://doi.org/10.7326/m18-2976
75. Brecheisen, R., Platel, B., ter Haar Romeny, B.M., Vilanova, A.: Illustrative uncertainty visualization of DTI fiber pathways. Vis. Comput. **29**(4), 297–309 (2013). https://doi.org/10.1007/S00371-012-0733-9
76. Brecheisen, R., Vilanova, A., Platel, B., ter Haar Romeny, B.: Parameter sensitivity visualization for DTI fiber tracking. IEEE Trans. Vis. Comput. Graph. **15**(6), 1441–1448 (2009). https://doi.org/10.1109/tvcg.2009.170
77. Brodlie, K., El-Khalili, N., Li, Y.: Using web-based computer graphics to teach surgery. Comput. Graph. **24**(1), 157–161 (2000). https://doi.org/10.1016/s0097-8493(99)00146-6
78. Brodlie, K., Wood, J.: Recent advances in volume visualization. Comput. Graph. Forum **20**(2), 125–148 (2001). https://doi.org/10.1111/1467-8659.00484
79. Bruckner, S.: Dynamic visibility-driven molecular surfaces. Comput. Graph. Forum **38**(2), 317–329 (2019). https://doi.org/10.1111/CGF.13640
80. Bruckner, S., Grimm, S., Kanitsar, A., Gröller, M.E.: Illustrative context-preserving volume rendering. In: Proceeding of EuroVis (2005). https://doi.org/10.2312/VisSym/EuroVis05/069-076
81. Bruckner, S., Gröller, E.: Enhancing depth-perception with flexible volumetric halos. IEEE Trans. Vis. Comput. Graph. **13**(6), 1344–1351 (2007). https://doi.org/10.1109/tvcg.2007.70555
82. Bruckner, S., Gröller, E.: Style transfer functions for illustrative volume rendering. Comput. Graph. Forum **26**(3), 715–724 (2007). https://doi.org/10.1111/J.1467-8659.2007.01095.X
83. Bruckner, S., Gröller, M.E.: VolumeShop: an interactive system for direct volume illustration. In: Proceeding of IEEE Visualization, pp. 671–678 (2005). https://doi.org/10.1109/VISUAL.2005.1532856
84. Bruckner, S., Šoltészová, V., Gröller, E., Hladuvka, J., Bühler, K., Jai, Y.Y., Dickson, B.J.: Braingazer-visual queries for neurobiology research. IEEE Trans. Vis. Comput. Graph. **15**(6), 1497–1504 (2009). https://doi.org/10.1109/tvcg.2009.121
85. Bryan, C., Guterman, G., Ma, K.L., Lewin, H., Larkin, D., Kim, J., Ma, J., Farre, M.: Synteny Explorer: an interactive visualization application for teaching genome evolution. IEEE Trans. Vis. Comput. Graph. **23**(1), 711–720 (2017). https://doi.org/10.1109/tvcg.2016.2598789
86. Bryan, J., Stredney, D., Wiet, G., Sessanna, D.: Virtual temporal bone dissection: a case study. In: Proceeding of IEEE Visualization, pp. 497–498 (2001). https://doi.org/10.1109/visual.2001.964561
87. Bryden, A., Phillips, G., Gleicher, M.: Automated illustration of molecular flexibility. IEEE Trans. Vis. Comput. Graph. **18**(1), 132–145 (2010). https://doi.org/10.1109/tvcg.2010.250
88. Budich, B., Garrison, L.A., Preim, B., Meuschke, M.: Reflections on AI-assisted character design for data-driven medical stories. In: Proceeding of Eurographics Workshop on Visual Computing for Biology and Medicine, pp. 87–91 (2023). https://doi.org/10.2312/vcbm.20231216
89. Buettner, R., Baumgartl, H., Konle, T., Haag, P.: A review of virtual reality and augmented reality literature in healthcare. In: Proceeding of IEEE Symposium on Industrial Electronics & Applications, pp. 1–6 (2020). https://doi.org/10.1109/ISIEA49364.2020.9188211
90. Bühler, K., Felkel, P., La Cruz, A.: Geometric methods for vessel visualization and quantification-a survey. In: Geometric Modeling For Scientific Visualization, pp. 399–419 (2004). https://doi.org/10.1007/978-3-662-07443-524
91. Byška, J., Le Muzic, M., Gröller, M.E., Viola, I., Kozlíková, B.: AnimoAminoMiner: exploration of protein tunnels and their properties in molecular dynamics. IEEE Trans. Vis. Comput. Graph. **22**(1), 747–756 (2016). https://doi.org/10.1109/tvcg.2015.2467434

92. Caballero, H.G., Corvó, A., van Meulen, F., Fonseca, P., Overeem, S., van Wijk, J.J., Westenberg, M.A.: PerSleep: a visual analytics approach for performance assessment of sleep staging models. In: Proceeding of Eurographics Workshop on Visual Computing in Biology and Medicine, pp. 123–133 (2021). https://doi.org/10.2312/VCBM.20211352
93. Cai, L.L., Nguyen, B.P., Chui, C.K., Ong, S.H.: Rule-enhanced transfer function generation for medical volume visualization. Comput. Graph. Forum **34**(3), 121–130 (2015). https://doi.org/10.1111/cgf.12624
94. Cai, Y., Lu, B., Fan, Z., Indhumathi, C., Lim, K.T., Chan, C.W., Jiang, Y., Li, L.: Bio-edutainment: learning life science through X gaming. Comput. Graph. **30**(1), 3–9 (2006). https://doi.org/10.1016/j.cag.2005.10.003
95. Cao, J., O'Day, D.R., Pliner, H.A., Kingsley, P.D., Deng, M., Daza, R.M., Zager, M.A., Aldinger, K.A., Blecher-Gonen, R., Zhang, F., Spielmann, M., Palis, J., Doherty, D., Steemers, F.J., Glass, I.A., Trapnell, C., Shendure, J.: A human cell atlas of fetal gene expression. Science **370**(6518) (2020). https://doi.org/10.1126/science.aba7721
96. Cedilnik, A., Baumes, J., Ibanez, L., Megason, S., Wylie, B.: Integration of information and volume visualization for analysis of cell lineage and gene expression during embryogenesis. In: Proceeding of Visualization and Data Analysis, vol. 6809, pp. 193–203 (2008). https://doi.org/10.1117/12.768014
97. ap Cenydd, L., John, N., Bloj, M., Walter, A., Phillips, N.: Visualizing the surface of a living human brain. IEEE Comput. Graph. Appl. **32**(2), 55–65 (2011). https://doi.org/10.1109/MCG.2011.105
98. Cercos-Pita, J.L., Cal, I., Duque, D., de Moreta, G.S.: NASAL-Geom, a free upper respiratory tract 3D model reconstruction software. Comput. Phys. Commun. **223**, 55–68 (2018). https://doi.org/10.1016/j.cpc.2017.10.008
99. Chaudhary, A., Jhaveri, S.J., Sanchez, A., Avila, L.S., Martin, K.M., Vacanti, A., Hanwell, M.D., Schroeder, W.: Cross-platform ubiquitous volume rendering using programmable shaders in VTK for scientific and medical visualization. IEEE Comput. Graph. Appl. **39**(1), 26–43 (2019). https://doi.org/10.1109/MCG.2018.2880818
100. Chen, D., Wax, M., Li, L., Liang, Z., Li, B., Kaufman, A.E.: A novel approach to extract colon lumen from CT images for virtual colonoscopy. IEEE Trans. Med. Imaging **19**(12), 1220–1226 (2000). https://doi.org/10.1109/42.897814
101. Chen, J., Roth, R.E., Naito, A.T., Lengerich, E.J., MacEachren, A.M.: Geovisual analytics to enhance spatial scan statistic interpretation: an analysis of us cervical cancer mortality. Int. J. Health Geogr. **7**(1), 57 (2008). https://doi.org/10.1186/1476-072X-7-57
102. Chen, K.H., Boettiger, A.N., Moffitt, J.R., Wang, S., Zhuang, X.: Spatially resolved, highly multiplexed RNA profiling in single cells. Science **348**(6233) (2015). https://doi.org/10.1126/science.aaa6090
103. Chen, L., Day, T.W., Tang, W., John, N.W.: Recent developments and future challenges in medical mixed reality. In: Proceeding of IEEE International Symposium on Mixed and Augmented Reality, pp. 123–135 (2017). https://doi.org/10.1109/ISMAR.2017.29
104. Chen, Z., An, S., Bai, X., Gong, F., Ma, L., Wan, L.: DensityPath: an algorithm to visualize and reconstruct cell state-transition path on density landscape for single-cell RNA sequencing data. Bioinformatics **35**(15), 2593–2601 (2018). https://doi.org/10.1093/bioinformatics/bty1009
105. Chheang, V., Apilla, V., Saalfeld, P., Boedecker, C., Huber, T., Huettl, F., Lang, H., Preim, B., Hansen, C.: Collaborative VR for liver surgery planning using wearable data gloves: An interactive demonstration. In: Proceeding of IEEE Conference on Virtual Reality and 3D User Interfaces—Abstracts and Workshops, pp. 768–768 (2021). https://doi.org/10.1109/VRW52623.2021.00268

106. Chheang, V., Saalfeld, P., Joeres, F., Boedecker, C., Huber, T., Huettl, F., Lang, H., Preim, B., Hansen, C.: A collaborative virtual reality environment for liver surgery planning. Comput. Graph. **99**, 234–246 (2021). https://doi.org/10.1016/j.cag.2021.07.009
107. Chi, E.H., Barry, P., Shoop, E., Carlis, J., Retzel, E., Riedl, J.: Visualization of biological sequence similarity search results. In: Proceeding of IEEE Visualization, pp. 44–51 (1995). https://doi.org/10.1109/VISUAL.1995.480794
108. Chi, E.H., Riedl, J., Shoop, E., Carlis, J., Retzel, E., Barry, P.: Flexible information visualization of multivariate data from biological sequence similarity searches. In: Proceeding of IEEE Visualization, pp. 133–140 (1996). https://doi.org/10.1109/VISUAL.1996.567796
109. Cipriano, G., Gleicher, M.: Molecular surface abstraction. IEEE Trans. Vis. Comput. Graph. **13**(6), 1608–1615 (2007). https://doi.org/10.1109/tvcg.2007.70578
110. Colaert, N., Helsens, K., Martens, L., Vandekerckhove, J., Gevaert, K.: Improved visualization of protein consensus sequences by iceLogo. Nat. Methods **6**(11), 786–787 (2009). https://doi.org/10.1038/nmeth1109-786
111. Coleman, R.G., Sharp, K.A.: Finding and characterizing tunnels in macromolecules with application to ion channels and pores. Biophys. J. **96**(2), 632–645 (2009). https://doi.org/10.1529/biophysj.108.135970
112. Coles, T.R., Meglan, D., John, N.W.: The role of haptics in medical training simulators: a survey of the state of the art. IEEE Trans. Haptics **4**(1), 51–66 (2010). https://doi.org/10.1109/toh.2010.19
113. Collins, T., Pizarro, D., Gasparini, S., Bourdel, N., Chauvet, P., Canis, M., Calvet, L., Bartoli, A.: Augmented reality guided laparoscopic surgery of the uterus. IEEE Trans. Med. Imaging **40**(1), 371–380 (2020). https://doi.org/10.1109/TMI.2020.3027442
114. Collura, T., Vuong, T.: An integrated computer graphics system for clinical EEG. In: Proceeding of IEEE Engineering in Medicine and Biology, pp. 1703–1704 (1989). https://doi.org/10.1109/iembs.1989.96415
115. Connolly, M.L.: Analytical molecular surface calculation. J. Appl. Crystallogr. **16**(5), 548–558 (1983). https://doi.org/10.1107/s0021889883010985
116. Correa, C., Ma, K.L.: Size-based transfer functions: a new volume exploration technique. IEEE Trans. Vis. Comput. Graph. **14**(6), 1380–1387 (2008). https://doi.org/10.1109/tvcg.2008.162
117. Correll, M., Ghosh, S., O'Connor, D., Gleicher, M.: Visualizing virus population variability from next generation sequencing data. In: Proceeding of IEEE Symposium on Biological Data Visualization, pp. 135–142 (2011). https://doi.org/10.1109/BioVis.2011.6094058
118. Corvò, A., Caballero, H.G., Westenberg, M.A., van Driel, M.A., van Wijk, J.J.: Visual analytics for hypothesis-driven exploration in computational pathology. IEEE Trans. Vis. Comput. Graph. **27**(10), 3851–3866 (2020). https://doi.org/10.1109/TVCG.2020.2990336
119. Corvò, A., van Driel, M.A., Westenberg, M.A.: PathoVA: A visual analytics tool for pathology diagnosis and reporting. In: Proceeding of IEEE Workshop on Visual Analytics in Healthcare, pp. 77–83 (2017). https://doi.org/10.1109/VAHC.2017.8387544
120. Corvò, A., Westenberg, M.A., van Driel, M.A., van Wijk, J.J.: PATHONE: from one thousand patients to one cell. In: Proceeding of Eurographics Workshop on Visual Computing in Biology and Medicine, pp. 111–115 (2016). https://doi.org/10.2312/VCBM.20161278
121. Corvò, A., Westenberg, M.A., van Driel, M.A., van Wijk, J.J.: Visual analytics in histopathology diagnostics: a protocol-based approach. In: Proceeding of Eurographics Workshop on Visual Computing for Biology and Medicine, pp. 23–32 (2018). https://doi.org/10.2312/vcbm.20181226
122. Corvò, A., Westenberg, M.A., Wimberger-Friedl, R., Fromme, S., Peeters, M.M.R., van Driel, M.A., van Wijk, J.J.: Visual analytics in digital pathology: challenges and opportunities. In: Proceeding of Eurographics Workshop on Visual Computing for Biology and Medicine, pp. 129–143 (2019). https://doi.org/10.2312/vcbm.20191240

123. Coto, E., Grimm, S., Bruckner, S., Gröller, E., Kanitsar, A., Rodriguez, O.: MammoExplorer: an advanced CAD application for breast DCE-MRI. In: Proceeding of Vision, Modelling, and Visualization, pp. 91–98 (2005)
124. Crippa, A., Maurits, N.M., Lorist, M.M., Roerdink, J.B.: Graph averaging as a means to compare multichannel EEG coherence networks and its application to the study of mental fatigue and neurodegenerative disease. Comput. Graph. **35**(2), 265–274 (2011). https://doi.org/10.1016/j.cag.2010.12.008
125. Cruz-Neira, C., Sandin, D.J., DeFanti, T.A., Kenyon, R.V., Hart, J.C.: The CAVE: audio visual experience automatic virtual environment. Commun. ACM **35**(6), 64–73 (1992). https://doi.org/10.1145/129888.129892
126. Cuellar-Partida, G., Renteria, M.E., MacGregor, S.: LocusTrack: Integrated visualization of GWAS results and genomic annotation. Source Code Biol. Med. **10**(1) (2015). https://doi.org/10.1186/s13029-015-0032-8
127. Cvek, U., Trutschl, M., Cannon, J.C., Scott, R.S., Rhoads, R.E.: 2D and 3D neural-network based visualization of high-dimensional biomedical data. In: Proceeding of IEEE Conference on Information Visualization (2007). https://doi.org/10.1109/iv.2007.5
128. Dappa, E., Higashigaito, K., Fornaro, J., Leschka, S., Wildermuth, S., Alkadhi, H.: Cinematic rendering-an alternative to volume rendering for 3D computed tomography imaging. Insights Imaging **7**(6), 849–856 (2016). https://doi.org/10.1007/s13244-016-0518-1
129. Darling, A.C., Mau, B., Blattner, F.R., Perna, N.T.: Mauve: multiple alignment of conserved genomic sequence with rearrangements. Genome Res. **14**(7), 1394–1403 (2004). https://doi.org/10.1101/gr.2289704
130. DeLano, W.L.: PyMol: an open-source molecular graphics tool. CCP4 Newsl. Protein Crystallogr. **40**, 82–92 (2002)
131. Delp, S.L., Loan, J.P., Basdogan, C., Buchanan, T., Rosen, J.: Surgical simulation: an emerging technology for military medical training. In: Proceeding of the National Forum: Military Telemedicine on-Line Today Research, Practice, and Opportunities, pp. 29–34 (1995). https://doi.org/10.1109/mtol.1995.504524
132. Detmer, F.J., Hettig, J., Schindele, D., Schostak, M., Hansen, C.: Virtual and augmented reality systems for renal interventions: a systematic review. IEEE Rev. Biomed. Eng. **10**, 78–94 (2017). https://doi.org/10.1109/rbme.2017.2749527
133. D'Hont, A., Denoeud, F., Aury, J.M., Baurens, F.C., Carreel, F., Garsmeur, O., Noel, B., Bocs, S., et al.: The banana (Musa acuminata) genome and the evolution of monocotyledonous plants. Nature **488**(7410), 213–217 (2012). https://doi.org/10.1038/nature11241
134. Dick, C., Georgii, J., Burgkart, R., Westermann, R.: Stress tensor field visualization for implant planning in orthopedics. IEEE Trans. Vis. Comput. Graph. **15**(6), 1399–1406 (2009). https://doi.org/10.1109/tvcg.2009.184
135. Diepenbrock, S., Praßni, J.S., Lindemann, F., Bothe, H.W., Ropinski, T.: Interactive planning for brain tumor resections. IEEE Comput. Graph. Appl. **31**(5), 6–13 (2011). https://doi.org/10.1109/mcg.2011.70
136. Diepenbrock, S., Praßni, J.S., Lindemann, F., Bothe, H.W., Ropinski, T.: Interactive visualization techniques for neurosurgery planning. In: Proceeding of Eurographics—Dirk Bartz Prize, pp. 13–16 (2011). https://doi.org/10.2312/EG2011/MED/013-016
137. Dietzsch, J., Heinrich, J., Nieselt, K., Bartz, D.: SpRay: A visual analytics approach for gene expression data. In: Proceeding of IEEE Symposium on Visual Analytics Science and Technology (2009). https://doi.org/10.1109/vast.2009.5333911
138. Dillenseger, J., Wendling, F.: Visualization of dynamic processes recorded during epileptic seizures. In: Proceeding of Eurographics—Short Papers, pp. 1–2 (1998). https://doi.org/10.2312/egs.19981003

139. Dinkla, K., Strobelt, H., Genest, B., Reiling, S., Borowsky, M., Pfister, H.: Screenit: visual analysis of cellular screens. IEEE Trans. Vis. Comput. Graph. **23**(1), 591–600 (2016). https://doi.org/10.1109/tvcg.2016.2598587
140. Dinkla, K., Westenberg, M.A., van Wijk, J.J.: Compressed adjacency matrices: untangling gene regulatory networks. IEEE Trans. Vis. Comput. Graph. **18**(12), 2457–2466 (2012). https://doi.org/10.1109/tvcg.2012.208
141. Dong, F., Clapworthy, G., Krokos, M.: Volume rendering of fine details within medical data. In: Proceeding of IEEE Visualization, pp. 387–577 (2001). https://doi.org/10.1109/VISUAL.2001.964537
142. Dong, F., Clapworthy, G., Lin, H., Krokos, M.: Nonphotorealistic rendering of medical volume data. IEEE Comput. Graph. Appl. **23**(4), 44–52 (2003). https://doi.org/10.1109/MCG.2003.1210864
143. Drebin, R.A., Carpenter, L., Hanrahan, P.: Volume rendering. ACM Siggraph Comput. Graph. **22**(4), 65–74 (1988). https://doi.org/10.1145/378456.378484
144. Drokhlyansky, E., Smillie, C.S., Wittenberghe, N.V., Ericsson, M., Griffin, G.K., Eraslan, G., Dionne, D., Cuoco, M.S., Goder-Reiser, M.N., Sharova, T., Kuksenko, O., Aguirre, A.J., Boland, G.M., Graham, D., Rozenblatt-Rosen, O., Xavier, R.J., Regev, A.: The human and mouse enteric nervous system at single-cell resolution. Cell **182**(6), 1606-1622.e23 (2020). https://doi.org/10.1016/j.cell.2020.08.003
145. Droste, P., Noack, S., Noh, K., Wiechert, W.: Customizable visualization of multi-omics data in the context of biochemical networks. In: Proceeding of IEEE Visualisation, pp. 21–25 (2009). https://doi.org/10.1109/viz.2009.22
146. Duran, D., Hermosilla, P., Ropinski, T., Kozlíková, B., Vinacua, À., Vázquez, P.: Visualization of large molecular trajectories. IEEE Trans. Vis. Comput. Graph. **25**(1), 987–996 (2019). https://doi.org/10.1109/TVCG.2018.2864851
147. Eagleson, R., Wucherer, P., Stefan, P., Duschko, Y., De Ribaupierre, S., Vollmar, C., Fallavollita, P., Navab, N.: Collaborative table-top VR display for neurosurgical planning. In: Proceeding of IEEE Virtual Reality, pp. 169–170 (2015). https://doi.org/10.1109/vr.2015.7223349
148. Edelsbrunner, H.: Deformable smooth surface design. Discrete Comput. Geom. **21**(1), 87–115 (1999). https://doi.org/10.1007/pl00009412
149. Eid, M., De Cecco, C.N., Nance, J.W., Jr., Caruso, D., Albrecht, M.H., Spandorfer, A.J., De Santis, D., Varga-Szemes, A., Schoepf, U.J.: Cinematic rendering in CT: a novel, lifelike 3D visualization technique. Am. J. Roentgenol. **209**(2), 370–379 (2017). https://doi.org/10.2214/AJR.17.17850
150. Engel, K., Hastreiter, P., Tomandl, B., Eberhardt, K., Ertl, T.: Combining local and remote visualization techniques for interactive volume rendering in medical applications. In: Proceeding of IEEE Visualization, pp. 449–452 (2000). https://doi.org/10.1109/VISUAL.2000.885729
151. Englund, R., Ropinski, T.: Quantitative and qualitative analysis of the perception of semi-transparent structures in direct volume rendering. Comput. Graph. Forum **37**(6), 174–187 (2018). https://doi.org/10.1111/cgf.13320
152. Ertl, T., Klein, T., Strengert, M., Kraus, M.: Adaptive sampling in three dimensions for volume rendering on GPUs. In: Proceeding of International Asia-Pacific Symposium on Visualization, pp. 113–120 (2007). https://doi.org/10.1109/APVIS.2007.329285
153. Eulzer, P., Meuschke, M., Mistelbauer, G., Lawonn, K.: Vessel maps: a survey of map-like visualizations of the cardiovascular system. Comput. Graph. Forum **41**(3), 645–673 (2022). https://doi.org/10.1111/cgf.14576
154. Evanko, D.: Supplement on visualizing biological data. Nat. Methods **7**(3), S1–S1 (2010). https://doi.org/10.1038/nmeth0310-S1

155. Ezquerra, N., Navazo, I., Morris, T.I., Monclus, E.: Graphics, vision, and visualization in medical imaging: a state of the art report. In: Proceeding of Eurographics—STARs (1999). https://doi.org/10.2312/egst.19991067
156. Falk, M., Krone, M., Ertl, T.: Atomistic visualization of mesoscopic whole-cell simulations using ray-casted instancing. Comput. Graph. Forum **32**(8), 195–206 (2013). https://doi.org/10.1111/CGF.12197
157. Falk, M., Ynnerman, A., Treanor, D., Lundström, C.: Interactive visualization of 3D histopathology in native resolution. IEEE Trans. Vis. Comput. Graph. **25**(1), 1008–1017 (2018). https://doi.org/10.1109/TVCG.2018.2864816
158. Fang, A., Sung, K., Pheng-Ann, H.: Interactive surface rendering for medical visualization. In: Proceeding of Graphics Interface, pp. 65–74 (1995). https://doi.org/10.20380/GI1995.08
159. Fang, Z., Moeller, T., Hamarneh, G., Celler, A.: Visualization and exploration of time-varying medical image data sets. In: Proceeding of Graphics Interface, pp. 281–288 (2007). https://doi.org/10.1145/1268517.1268563
160. Feng, D., Whitehurst, C.E., Shan, D., Hill, J.D., Yue, Y.G.: Single cell explorer, collaboration-driven tools to leverage large-scale single cell RNA-seq data. BMC Genomics **20**(1) (2019). https://doi.org/10.1186/s12864-019-6053-y
161. Fjeld, M., Voegtli, B.M.: Augmented chemistry: an interactive educational workbench. In: Proceeding of International Symposium on Mixed and Augmented Reality, pp. 259–266 (2002). https://doi.org/10.1109/ismar.2002.1115100
162. Floricel, C., Nipu, N., Biggs, M., Wentzel, A., Canahuate, G., Van Dijk, L., Mohamed, A., Fuller, C.D., Marai, G.E.: THALIS: human-machine analysis of longitudinal symptoms in cancer therapy. IEEE Trans. Vis. Comput. Graph. **28**(1), 151–161 (2021). https://doi.org/10.1109/tvcg.2021.3114810
163. Fonseca, T.C.F., Campos, T.P.R.: SOFT-RT: software for IMRT simulations based on MCNPx code. Appl. Radiat. Isot. **117**, 111–117 (2016). https://doi.org/10.1016/j.apradiso.2015.12.061
164. Fotouhi, J., Mehrfard, A., Song, T., Johnson, A., Osgood, G., Unberath, M., Armand, M., Navab, N.: Development and pre-clinical analysis of spatiotemporal-aware augmented reality in orthopedic interventions. IEEE Trans. Med. Imaging **40**(2), 765–778 (2020). https://doi.org/10.1109/tmi.2020.3037013
165. Fritsch, J.M., Ellis, R.A., Jacobi, T.H., Marshall, G.R.: A macromodular graphics system for protein structure research. Comput. Graph. **1**(2–3), 271–278 (1975). https://doi.org/10.1016/0097-8493(75)90018-7
166. Fung, D.C.Y., Hong, S.H., Koschützki, D., Schreiber, F., Xu, K.: Visual analysis of overlapping biological networks. In: Proceeding of Information Visualisation (2009). https://doi.org/10.1109/iv.2009.55
167. Furmanová, K., Grossmann, N., Muren, L.P., Casares-Magaz, O., Moiseenko, V., Einck, J.P., Gröller, M.E., Raidou, R.G.: VAPOR: visual analytics for the exploration of pelvic organ variability in radiotherapy. Comput. Graph. **91**, 25–38 (2020). https://doi.org/10.1016/j.cag.2020.07.001
168. Furmanová, K., Jurčík, A., Kozlíková, B., Hauser, H., Byška, J.: Multiscale visual drilldown for the analysis of large ensembles of multi-body protein complexes. IEEE Trans. Vis. Comput. Graph. **26**(1), 843–852 (2020). https://doi.org/10.1109/tvcg.2019.2934333
169. Furmanová, K., Muren, L.P., Casares-Magaz, O., Moiseenko, V., Einck, J.P., Pilskog, S., Raidou, R.G.: PREVIS: predictive visual analytics of anatomical variability for radiotherapy decision support. Comput. Graph. **97**, 126–138 (2021). https://doi.org/10.1016/j.cag.2021.04.010
170. Furmanová, K., Vávra, O., Kozlíková, B., Damborský, J., Vonásek, V., Bednář, D., Byška, J.: DockVis: visual analysis of molecular docking trajectories. Comput. Graph. Forum **39**(6), 452–464 (2020). https://doi.org/10.1111/CGF.14048

171. Galea, M.D.: Telemedicine in rehabilitation. Phys. Med. Rehabil. Clin. **30**(2), 473–483 (2019). https://doi.org/10.1016/j.pmr.2018.12.002
172. Ganglberger, F., Swoboda, N., Frauenstein, L., Kaczanowska, J., Haubensak, W., Bühler, K.: BrainTrawler: a visual analytics framework for iterative exploration of heterogeneous big brain data. Comput. Graph. **82**, 304–320 (2019). https://doi.org/10.1016/j.cag.2019.05.032
173. Garcia Caballero, H.S., Westenberg, M.A., Gebre, B., van Wijk, J.J.: V-Awake: a visual analytics approach for correcting sleep predictions from deep learning models. Comput. Graph. Forum **38**(3), 1–12 (2019). https://doi.org/10.1111/CGF.13667
174. Gardeux, V., David, F.P.A., Shajkofci, A., Schwalie, P.C., Deplancke, B.: ASAP: a web-based platform for the analysis and interactive visualization of single-cell RNA-seq data. Bioinformatics **33**(19), 3123–3125 (2017). https://doi.org/10.1093/bioinformatics/btx337
175. Garrison, L.A., Kolesar, I., Viola, I., Hauser, H., Bruckner, S.: Trends & opportunities in visualization for physiology: a multiscale overview. Comput. Graph. Forum **41**(3), 609–643 (2022). https://doi.org/10.1111/CGF.14575
176. Gassen, S.V., Callebaut, B., Helden, M.J.V., Lambrecht, B.N., Demeester, P., Dhaene, T., Saeys, Y.: FlowSOM: using self-organizing maps for visualization and interpretation of cytometry data. Cytometry A **87**(7), 636–645 (2015). https://doi.org/10.1002/cyto.a.22625
177. Gasteiger, R., Neugebauer, M., Beuing, O., Preim, B.: The FLOWLENS: a focus-and-context visualization approach for exploration of blood flow in cerebral aneurysms. IEEE Trans. Vis. Comput. Graph. **17**(12), 2183–2192 (2011). https://doi.org/10.1109/tvcg.2011.243
178. Gasteiger, R., Neugebauer, M., Kubisch, C., Preim, B.: Adapted surface visualization of cerebral aneurysms with embedded blood flow information. In: Proceeding of Eurographics Workshop on Visual Computing in Biology and Medicine, pp. 25–32 (2010). https://doi.org/10.2312/VCBM/VCBM10/025-032
179. Gawron, P., Ostaszewski, M., Satagopam, V., Gebel, S., Mazein, A., Kuzma, M., Zorzan, S., McGee, F., Otjacques, B., Balling, R., Schneider, R.: MINERVA—a platform for visualization and curation of molecular interaction networks. npj Syst. Biol. Appl. **2**(1), 1–6 (2016). https://doi.org/10.1038/npjsba.2016.20
180. Gear, J.I., Cummings, C., Craig, A.J., Divoli, A., Long, C.D., Tapner, M., Flux, G.D.: Abdo-Man: a 3D-printed anthropomorphic phantom for validating quantitative SIRT. EJNMMI Phys. **3**(1), 1–16 (2016). https://doi.org/10.1186/s40658-016-0151-6
181. Gehlenborg, N., O'Donoghue, S.I., Baliga, N.S., Goesmann, A., Hibbs, M.A., Kitano, H., Kohlbacher, O., Neuweger, H., Schneider, R., Tenenbaum, D., Gavin, A.C.: Visualization of omics data for systems biology. Nat. Methods **7**(S3), S56–S68 (2010). https://doi.org/10.1038/nmeth.1436
182. George, G., Gan, S., Huang, Y., Appleby, P., Nar, A.S., Venkatesan, R., Mohan, V., Palmer, C.N.A., Doney, A.S.F.: PheGWAS: a new dimension to visualize GWAS across multiple phenotypes. Bioinformatics **36**(8), 2500–2505 (2019). https://doi.org/10.1093/bioinformatics/btz944
183. Georgii, J., von Dresky, C., Meier, S., Demedts, D., Schumann, C., Preusser, T., Bender, J., Erleben, K., Galin, E.: Focused ultrasound-efficient GPU simulation methods for therapy planning. In: Proceeding of VRIPHYS, pp. 119–128 (2011). https://doi.org/10.2312/PE/VRIPHYS/VRIPHYS11/119-128
184. Gershon, N., Cappelletti, J., Hinds, S., Glenn, M.: Image understanding, visualization, and registration of magnetic resonance (MR) and positron emission tomography (PET) images. In: Proceeding of IEEE Engineering in Medicine and Biology, pp. 1295–1296 (1990). https://doi.org/10.1109/IEMBS.1990.691757
185. Gevins, A.S., Yeager, C.L., Diamond, S.L.: Interactive analysis and display of the electroencephalogram (EEG) in real time. Comput. Graph. **1**(4), 329–335 (1975). https://doi.org/10.1016/0097-8493(75)90048-5

186. Ghods, A., Caffrey, K., Lin, B., Fraga, K., Fritz, R., Schmitter-Edgecombe, M., Hundhausen, C., Cook, D.J.: Iterative design of visual analytics for a clinician-in-the-loop smart home. IEEE J. Biomed. Health Inform. **23**(4), 1742–1748 (2018). https://doi.org/10.1109/JBHI.2018.2864287
187. Gibson, S.F.: Constrained elastic surface nets: Generating smooth surfaces from binary segmented data. In: Proceeding of Medical Image Computing and Computer-Assisted Intervention, pp. 888–898 (1998). https://doi.org/10.1007/bfb0056277
188. Giesen, C., Wang, H.A.O., Schapiro, D., Zivanovic, N., Jacobs, A., Hattendorf, B., Schüffler, P.J., Grolimund, D., Buhmann, J.M., Brandt, S., Varga, Z., Wild, P.J., Günther, D., Bodenmiller, B.: Highly multiplexed imaging of tumor tissues with subcellular resolution by mass cytometry. Nat. Methods **11**(4), 417–422 (2014). https://doi.org/10.1038/nmeth.2869
189. Gillet, A., Sanner, M., Stoffler, D., Olson, A.: Tangible interfaces for structural molecular biology. Structure **13**(3), 483–491 (2005). https://doi.org/10.1016/j.str.2005.01.009
190. Gillies, D., Williams, C.: An interactive graphic simulator for the teaching of fibrendoscopic techniques. In: Proceeding of Eurographics—Technical Papers (1987). https://doi.org/10.2312/egtp.19871010
191. Gillmann, C., Saur, D., Wischgoll, T., Scheuermann, G.: Uncertainty-aware visualization in medical imaging-a survey. Comput. Graph. Forum **40**(3), 665–689 (2021). https://doi.org/10.1111/cgf.14333
192. Gillmann, C., Smit, N.N., Gröller, E., Preim, B., Vilanova, A., Wischgoll, T.: Ten open challenges in medical visualization. IEEE Comput. Graph. Appl. **41**(5), 7–15 (2021). https://doi.org/10.1109/mcg.2021.3094858
193. Gisbrecht, A., Hammer, B., Mokbel, B., Sczyrba, A.: Nonlinear dimensionality reduction for cluster identification in metagenomic samples. In: Proceeding of Information Visualisation (2013). https://doi.org/10.1109/iv.2013.22
194. Glaser, J.R., Glaser, E.M.: Neuron imaging with neurolucida-a PC-based system for image combining microscopy. Comput. Med. Imaging Graph. **14**(5), 307–317 (1990). https://doi.org/10.1016/0895-6111(90)90105-k
195. Glaßer, S., Oeltze, S., Hennemuth, A., Kubisch, C., Mahnken, A., Wilhelmsen, S., Preim, B.: Automatic transfer function specification for visual emphasis of coronary artery plaque. Comput. Graph. Forum **29**(1), 191–201 (2010). https://doi.org/10.1111/J.1467-8659.2009.01590.X
196. Glaßer, S., Preim, U., Tönnies, K., Preim, B.: A visual analytics approach to diagnosis of breast DCE-MRI data. Comput. Graph. **34**(5), 602–611 (2010). https://doi.org/10.1016/j.cag.2010.05.016
197. Goldau, M., Wiebel, A., Gorbach, N.S., Melzer, C., Hlawitschka, M., Scheuermann, G., Tittgemeyer, M.: Fiber stippling: an illustrative rendering for probabilistic diffusion tractography. In: Proceeding of IEEE Symposium on Biological Data Visualization, pp. 23–30 (2011). https://doi.org/10.1109/biovis.2011.6094044
198. Goodsell, D.S., Dutta, S., Voigt, M., Zardecki, C.: Molecular storytelling for online structural biology outreach and education. Struct. Dyn. **8**(2) (2021). https://doi.org/10.1063/4.0000077
199. Grace, C., Farrall, M., Watkins, H., Goel, A.: Manhattan++: displaying genome-wide association summary statistics with multiple annotation layers. BMC Bioinformatics **20**(1), 610 (2019). https://doi.org/10.1186/s12859-019-3201-y
200. Grimson, W.E.L., Ettinger, G.J., White, S.J., Lozano-Perez, T., Wells, W., Kikinis, R.: An automatic registration method for frameless stereotaxy, image guided surgery, and enhanced reality visualization. IEEE Trans. Med. Imaging **15**(2), 129–140 (1996). https://doi.org/10.1109/42.491415
201. Gschwandtner, T., Aigner, W., Kaiser, K., Miksch, S., Seyfang, A.: CareCruiser: exploring and visualizing plans, events, and effects interactively. In: Proceeding of IEEE Pacific Visualization Symposium, pp. 43–50 (2011). https://doi.org/10.1109/pacificvis.2011.5742371

202. Gu, Z., Eils, R., Schlesner, M.: HilbertCurve: an R/Bioconductor package for high-resolution visualization of genomic data. Bioinformatics **32**(15), 2372–2374 (2016). https://doi.org/10.1093/bioinformatics/btw161
203. Guan, S.Y.: Guided image interpretation in neuroanatomy. Ph.D. thesis, Texas A&M University (1991)
204. Günther, T., Poliwoda, C., Reinhart, C., Hesser, J., Männer, R., Meinzer, H.P., Baur, H.I.: VIRIM: a massively parallel processor for real-time volume visualization in medicine. In: Proceeding of Eurographics Workshop on Graphics Hardware, pp. 103–108 (1994). https://doi.org/10.2312/EGGH/EGGH94/103-108
205. Haase, H., Strassner, J., Dai, F.: VR techniques for the investigation of molecule data. Comput. Graph. **20**(2), 207–217 (1996). https://doi.org/10.1016/0097-8493(95)00127-1
206. Hadwiger, M., Beyer, J., Jeong, W.K., Pfister, H.: Interactive volume exploration of petascale microscopy data streams using a visualization-driven virtual memory approach. IEEE Trans. Vis. Comput. Graph. **18**(12), 2285–2294 (2012). https://doi.org/10.1109/tvcg.2012.240
207. Hahn, H.K., Preim, B., Selle, D., Peitgen, H.O.: Visualization and interaction techniques for the exploration of vascular structures. In: Proceeding of IEEE Visualization, pp. 395–578 (2001). https://doi.org/10.1109/visual.2001.964538
208. Hakone, A., Harrison, L., Ottley, A., Winters, N., Gutheil, C., Han, P.K., Chang, R.: PROACT: iterative design of a patient-centered visualization for effective prostate cancer health risk communication. IEEE Trans. Vis. Comput. Graph. **23**(1), 601–610 (2016). https://doi.org/10.1109/tvcg.2016.2598588
209. Halier, S., Angenent, S., Tannenbaurn, A., Kikinis, R.: Nondistorting flattening maps and the 3-D visualization of colon CT images. IEEE Trans. Med. Imaging **19**(7), 665–670 (2000). https://doi.org/10.1109/42.875181
210. Halladjian, S., Kouřil, D., Miao, H., Gröller, M.E., Viola, I., Isenberg, T.: Multiscale unfolding: illustratively visualizing the whole genome at a glance. IEEE Trans. Vis. Comput. Graph. **28**(10), 3456–3470 (2022). https://doi.org/10.1109/TVCG.2021.3065443
211. Halladjian, S., Miao, H., Kouřil, D., Gröller, M.E., Viola, I., Isenberg, T.: Scale trotter: illustrative visual travels across negative scales. IEEE Trans. Vis. Comput. Graph. **26**(1), 654–664 (2019). https://doi.org/10.1109/tvcg.2019.2934334
212. Halle, M., Demeusy, V., Kikinis, R.: The open anatomy browser: a collaborative web-based viewer for interoperable anatomy atlases. Front. Neuroinform. **11**, 22 (2017). https://doi.org/10.3389/fninf.2017.00022
213. Hamdan, I., Bert, J., Rest, C.C.L., Tasu, J.P., Boussion, N., Valeri, A., Dardenne, G., Visvikis, D.: Fully automatic deformable registration of pretreatment MRI/CT for image-guided prostate radiotherapy planning. Med. Phys. **44**(12), 6447–6455 (2017). https://doi.org/10.1002/mp.12629
214. Hamilton, N.A., Wang, J.T., Kerr, M.C., Teasdale, R.D.: Statistical and visual differentiation of subcellular imaging. BMC Bioinformatics **10**(1), 1–12 (2009). https://doi.org/10.1186/1471-2105-10-94
215. Hansen, C., Köhn, A., Zidowitz, S., Peitgen, H.O., Ritter, F.: Simultaneous visualization of preoperative planning models and intraoperative 2D ultrasound for liver surgery. In: Proceeding of Eurographics—Short Papers, pp. 73–76 (2007). https://doi.org/10.2312/EGS.20071037
216. Hansen, C., Wieferich, J., Ritter, F., Rieder, C., Peitgen, H.O.: Illustrative visualization of 3D planning models for augmented reality in liver surgery. Int. J. Comput. Assist. Radiol. Surg. **5**(2), 133–141 (2010). https://doi.org/10.1007/S11548-009-0365-3
217. Hansen, C., Zidowitz, S., Preim, B., Stavrou, G., Oldhafer, K.J., Hahn, H.K.: Impact of model-based risk analysis for liver surgery planning. Int. J. Comput. Assist. Radiol. Surg. **9**(3), 473–480 (2014). https://doi.org/10.1007/s11548-013-0937-0

218. Hansen, M., Meads, D., Pang, A.: Comparative visualization of protein structure-sequence alignments. In: Proceeding of IEEE Symposium on Information Visualization, pp. 106–110 (1998). https://doi.org/10.1109/INFVIS.1998.729566
219. Harvey, E., Gingold, C.: Haptic representation of the atom. In: Proceeding of IEEE Conference on Information Visualization, pp. 232–235 (2000). https://doi.org/10.1109/iv.2000.859761
220. Hastreiter, P., Rezk-Salama, C., Tomandl, B., Eberhardt, K.E.W., Ertl, T.: Fast analysis of intracranical aneurysms based on interactive direct volume rendering and CTA. In: Proceeding of Medical Image Computing and Computer-Assisted Intervention, pp. 660–669 (1998). https://doi.org/10.1007/bfb0056252
221. Hauser, H., Mroz, L., Bischi, G.I., Gröller, M.E.: Two-level volume rendering. IEEE Trans. Vis. Comput. Graph. **7**(3), 242–252 (2001). https://doi.org/10.1109/2945.942692
222. Heckel, F., Moltz, J.H., Tietjen, C., Hahn, H.K.: Sketch-based editing tools for tumour segmentation in 3D medical images. Comput. Graph. Forum **32**(8), 144–157 (2013). https://doi.org/10.1111/CGF.12193
223. Heinrich, F., Huettl, F., Schmidt, G., Paschold, M., Kneist, W., Huber, T., Hansen, C.: HoloPointer: a virtual augmented reality pointer for laparoscopic surgery training. Int. J. Comput. Assist. Radiol. Surg. **16**(1), 161–168 (2021). https://doi.org/10.1007/S11548-020-02272-2
224. Heinrich, J., Vehlow, C., Battke, F., Jäger, G., Weiskopf, D., Nieselt, K.: iHAT: interactive hierarchical aggregation table for genetic association data. BMC Bioinformatics **13**(S8), S2 (2012). https://doi.org/10.1186/1471-2105-13-S8-S2
225. Hennig, A., Bernhardt, J., Nieselt, K.: Pan-Tetris: an interactive visualisation for Pan-genomes. BMC Bioinformatics **16**(S11) (2015). https://doi.org/10.1186/1471-2105-16-s11-s3
226. Herghelegiu, P.C., Manta, V., Perin, R., Bruckner, S., Gröller, E.: Biopsy planner-visual analysis for needle pathway planning in deep seated brain tumor biopsy. Comput. Graph. Forum **31**(3), 1085–1094 (2012). https://doi.org/10.1111/J.1467-8659.2012.03101.X
227. Hermosilla, P., Guallar, V., Vinacua, À., Vázquez, P.P.: Instant visualization of secondary structures of molecular models. In: Proceeding of the Eurographics Workshop on Visual Computing for Biology and Medicine, pp. 51–60 (2015). https://doi.org/10.2312/VCBM.20151208
228. Hermosilla, P., Guallar, V., Vinacua, A., Vázquez, P.P.: High quality illustrative effects for molecular rendering. Comput. Graph. **54**, 113–120 (2016). https://doi.org/10.1016/j.cag.2015.07.017
229. Hermosilla, P., Maisch, S., Vázquez Alcocer, P.P., Ropinski, T.: Improving perception of molecular surface visualizations by incorporating translucency effects. In: Proceeding of Eurographics Workshop on Visual Computing for Biology and Medicine, pp. 185–195 (2018). https://doi.org/10.2312/VCBM.20181244
230. Hermosilla, P., Vázquez, P., Vinacua, A., Ropinski, T.: A general illumination model for molecular visualization. Comput. Graph. Forum **37**(3), 367–378 (2018). https://doi.org/10.1111/CGF.13426
231. Hess, M., Jente, D., Wiemeyer, J., Hamacher, K., Goesele, M.: Visual analysis and comparison of multiple sequence alignments. In: Proceeding of Eurographics Workshop on Visual Computing for Biology and Medicine (2016). https://doi.org/10.2312/vcbm.20161268
232. Hibbs, M., Wallace, G., Dunham, M., Li, K., Troyanskaya, O.: Viewing the larger context of genomic data through horizontal integration. In: Proceeding of IEEE Conference on Information Visualization (2007). https://doi.org/10.1109/iv.2007.120
233. Higuera, F.V., Sauber, N., Tomandl, B., Nimsky, C., Greiner, G., Hastreiter, P.: Automatic adjustment of bidimensional transfer functions for direct volume visualization of intracranial aneurysms. In: Proceeding of SPIE Medical Imaging: Visualization, Image-Guided Procedures, and Display, vol. 5367, pp. 275–284 (2004). https://doi.org/10.1117/12.535534

234. Hladuvka, J., König, A., Gröller, E.: Curvature-based transfer functions for direct volume rendering. In: Proceeding of Spring Conference on Computer Graphics, vol. 16-5, pp. 58–65 (2000)
235. Ho, J.W.K., Manwaring, T., Hong, S.H., Roehm, U., Fung, D.C.Y., Xu, K., Kraska, T., Hart, D.: PathBank: Web-based querying and visualziation of an integrated biological pathway database. In: Proceeding of Computer Graphics, Imaging and Visualisation, pp. 84–89 (2006). https://doi.org/10.1109/cgiv.2006.70
236. Hodges, L.F., Rothbaum, B.: Virtually Better virtual reality system. CyberPsychol. Behav. **1**(4), 405–409 (1998). https://doi.org/10.1089/CPB.1998.1.405
237. Hoffman, H.G., Doctor, J.N., Patterson, D.R., Carrougher, G.J., Furness, T.A., III.: Virtual reality as an adjunctive pain control during burn wound care in adolescent patients. Pain **85**(1–2), 305–309 (2000). https://doi.org/10.1016/s0304-3959(99)00275-4
238. Hoffman, P., Grinstein, G., Marx, K., Grosse, I., Stanley, E.: DNA visual and analytic data mining. In: Proceeding of IEEE Visualization, pp. 437–442 (1997). https://doi.org/10.1109/visual.1997.663916
239. Höhne, K.H., Bernstein, R.: Shading 3D-images from CT using gray-level gradients. IEEE Trans. Med. Imaging **5**(1), 45–47 (1986). https://doi.org/10.1109/tmi.1986.4307738
240. Höhne, K.H., Bomans, M., Pommert, A., Riemer, M., Schiers, C., Tiede, U., Wiebecke, G.: 3D-visualization of tomographic volume data using the generalized voxel-model. In: Proceeding of Chapel Hill Workshop on Volume Visualization, pp. 51–57 (1989). https://doi.org/10.1145/329129.329364
241. Höhne, K.H., Bomans, M., Riemer, M., Schubert, R., Tiede, U., Lierse, W.: A volume-based anatomical atlas. IEEE Comput. Graph. Appl. **12**(04), 73–77 (1992). https://doi.org/10.1109/38.144829
242. Holden, M., Todorov, E., Callahan, J., Bizzi, E.: Virtual environment training improves motor performance in two patients with stroke: case report. J. Neurol. Phys. Ther. **23**(2), 57–67 (1999)
243. Höllt, T., Pezzotti, N., van Unen, V., Koning, F., Eisemann, E., Lelieveldt, B., Vilanova, A.: Cytosplore: interactive immune cell phenotyping for large single-cell datasets. Comput. Graph. Forum **35**(3), 171–180 (2016). https://doi.org/10.1111/cgf.12893
244. Höllt, T., Pezzotti, N., van Unen, V., Koning, F., Lelieveldt, B.P., Vilanova, A.: CyteGuide: visual guidance for hierarchical single-cell analysis. IEEE Trans. Vis. Comput. Graph. **24**(1), 739–748 (2018). https://doi.org/10.1109/tvcg.2017.2744318
245. Höllt, T., Pezzotti, N., van Unen, V., Li, N., Koning, F., Eisemann, E., Lelieveldt, B.P.F., Vilanova, A.: Cytosplore: Interactive visual single-cell profiling of the immune system. In: Proceeding of Eurographics—Dirk Bartz Prize (2019). https://doi.org/10.2312/egm.20191032
246. Hong, L., Kaufman, A., Wei, Y.C., Viswambharan, A., Wax, M., Liang, Z.: 3D virtual colonoscopy. In: Proceeding of Biomedical Visualization, pp. 26–32 (1995). https://doi.org/10.1109/biovis.1995.528702
247. Hong, M.K., Lakshmi, U., Olson, T.A., Wilcox, L.: Visual ODLs: Co-designing patient-generated observations of daily living to support data-driven conversations in pediatric care. In: Proceeding of the CHI Conference on Human Factors in Computing Systems, pp. 1–13 (2018). https://doi.org/10.1145/3173574.3174050
248. Hong, W., Qiu, F., Kaufmann, A.: A pipeline for computer aided polyp detection. IEEE Trans. Vis. Comput. Graph. **12**(5), 861–868 (2006). https://doi.org/10.1109/tvcg.2006.112
249. Honigmann, D., Ruisz, J., Haider, C.: Adaptive design of a global opacity transfer function for direct volume rendering of ultrasound data. In: Proceeding of IEEE Visualization, pp. 489–496 (2003). https://doi.org/10.1109/VISUAL.2003.1250411
250. Hotz, I., Sreevalsan-Nair, J., Hagen, H., Hamann, B.: Tensor field reconstruction based on eigenvector and eigenvalue interpolation. In: Dagstuhl Follow-Ups, vol. 1 (2010). https://doi.org/10.4230/dfu.sciviz.2010.110

251. Huang, H., Wang, Y., Rudin, C., Browne, E.P.: Towards a comprehensive evaluation of dimension reduction methods for transcriptomic data visualization. Commun. Biol. **5**(1) (2022). https://doi.org/10.1038/s42003-022-03628-x
252. Huisman, S.M., van Lew, B., Mahfouz, A., Pezzotti, N., Höllt, T., Michielsen, L., Vilanova, A., Reinders, M.J., Lelieveldt, B.P.: BrainScope: interactive visual exploration of the spatial and temporal human brain transcriptome. Nucleic Acids Res., e83 (2017). https://doi.org/10.1093/nar/gkx046
253. Huntsberger, T., Peroni, M., Augustine, J.: Volumetric modeling of neuronal populations. In: Proceeding of Visualization in Biomedical Computing, pp. 36–37 (1990). https://doi.org/10.1109/vbc.1990.109299
254. Hurdal, M.K., Kurtz, K.W., Banks, D.C.: Case study: interacting with cortical flat maps of the human brain. In: Proceeding of IEEE Visualization, pp. 469–472 (2001). https://doi.org/10.1109/VISUAL.2001.964553
255. Interrante, V., Fuchs, H., Pizer, S.: Enhancing transparent skin surfaces with ridge and valley lines. In: Proceeding of IEEE Visualization, pp. 52–59 (1995). https://doi.org/10.1109/visual.1995.480795
256. Interrante, V., Fuchs, H., Pizer, S.: Illustrating transparent surfaces with curvature-directed strokes. In: Proceeding of IEEE Visualization, pp. 211–218 (1996). https://doi.org/10.1109/visual.1996.568110
257. Interrante, V., Fuchs, H., Pizer, S.M.: Conveying the 3D shape of smoothly curving transparent surfaces via texture. IEEE Trans. Vis. Comput. Graph. **3**(2), 98–117 (1997). https://doi.org/10.1109/2945.597794
258. Isenberg, T., Isenberg, P., Chen, J., Sedlmair, M., Möller, T.: A systematic review on the practice of evaluating visualization. IEEE Trans. Vis. Comput. Graph. **19**(12), 2818–2827 (2013)
259. Jaffe, D.L., Brown, D.A., Pierson-Carey, C.D., Buckley, E.L., Lew, H.L.: Stepping over obstacles to improve walking in individuals with poststroke hemiplegia. J. Rehabil. Res. Dev. **41**(3aA), 283–92 (2004). https://doi.org/10.1682/jrrd.2004.03.0283
260. Jainek, W.M., Born, S., Bartz, D., Straßer, W., Fischer, J.: Illustrative hybrid visualization and exploration of anatomical and functional brain data. Comput. Graph. Forum **27**(3), 855–862 (2008). https://doi.org/10.1111/J.1467-8659.2008.01217.X
261. Jankun-Kelly, T., Lindeman, A.D., Bridges, S.M.: Exploratory visual analysis of conserved domains on multiple sequence alignments. BMC Bioinformatics **10**(S11), S7 (2009). https://doi.org/10.1186/1471-2105-10-s11-s7
262. Janssen, S., de Ruyter van Steveninck, J., Salim, H.S., Cockx, H.M., Bloem, B.R., Heida, T., Van Wezel, R.J.: The effects of augmented reality visual cues on turning in place in Parkinson's disease patients with freezing of gait. Front. Neurol. **11**, 185 (2020). https://doi.org/10.3389/fneur.2020.00185
263. Jeong, S.J., Kaufman, A.E.: Interactive wireless virtual colonoscopy. Vis. Comput. **23**(8), 545–557 (2007). https://doi.org/10.1007/s00371-007-0117-8
264. Jeong, W.K., Beyer, J., Hadwiger, M., Blue, R., Law, C., Vázquez-Reina, A., Reid, R.C., Lichtman, J., Pfister, H.: Ssecrett and neurotrace: interactive visualization and analysis tools for large-scale neuroscience data sets. IEEE Comput. Graph. Appl. **30**(3), 58–70 (2010). https://doi.org/10.1109/mcg.2010.56
265. Jeong, W.K., Schneider, J., Turney, S., Faulkner-Jones, B.E., Meyer, D., Westermann, R., Reid, R.C., Lichtman, J., Pfister, H.: Interactive histology of large-scale biomedical image stacks. IEEE Trans. Vis. Comput. Graph. **16**(6), 1386–1395 (2010). https://doi.org/10.1109/tvcg.2010.168
266. Ji, C., van de Gronde, J.J., Maurits, N.M., Roerdink, J.B.: Visual exploration of dynamic multichannel EEG coherence networks. Comput. Graph. Forum **38**(1), 507–520 (2019). https://doi.org/10.1111/cgf.13588

267. Ji, C., Maurits, N.M., Roerdink, J.B.: Visual analysis of evolution of EEG coherence networks employing temporal multidimensional scaling. In: Proceeding of Eurographics Workshop on Visual Computing in Biology and Medicine, pp. 95–99 (2018). https://doi.org/10.2312/VCBM.20181233
268. Jianu, R., Demiralp, C., Laidlaw, D.: Exploring 3D DTI fiber tracts with linked 2D representations. IEEE Trans. Vis. Comput. Graph. **15**(6), 1449–1456 (2009). https://doi.org/10.1109/tvcg.2009.141
269. Jianu, R., Demiralp, C., Laidlaw, D.H.: Exploring brain connectivity with two-dimensional neural maps. IEEE Trans. Vis. Comput. Graph. **18**(6), 978–987 (2011). https://doi.org/10.1109/TVCG.2011.82
270. Jin, Z., Cui, S., Guo, S., Gotz, D., Sun, J., Cao, N.: CarePre: an intelligent clinical decision assistance system. ACM Trans. Comput. Healthc. **1**(1), 1–20 (2020). https://doi.org/10.1145/3344258
271. Joeres, F., Black, D., Razavizadeh, S., Hansen, C.: Audiovisual AR concepts for laparoscopic subsurface structure navigation. In: Proceeding of Graphics Interface, pp. 224–230 (2021). https://doi.org/10.20380/GI2021.34
272. Johnson, C.K.: OR TEP-II: a FORTRAN thermal-ellipsoid plot program for crystal structure illustrations. Technical report, Oak Ridge National Lab (1976)
273. Johnson, G.T., Autin, L., Al-Alusi, M., Goodsell, D.S., Sanner, M.F., Olson, A.J.: cellPACK: a virtual mesoscope to model and visualize structural systems biology. Nat. Methods **12**(1), 85–91 (2015). https://doi.org/10.1038/nmeth.3204
274. Johnston, A.P., Rae, J., Ariotti, N., Bailey, B., Lilja, A., Webb, R., Ferguson, C., Maher, S., Davis, T.P., Webb, R.I., et al.: Journey to the centre of the cell: virtual reality immersion into scientific data. Traffic **19**(2), 105–110 (2018). https://doi.org/10.1111/tra.12538
275. Jones, T.R., Kang, I.H., Wheeler, D.B., Lindquist, R.A., Papallo, A., Sabatini, D.M., Golland, P., Carpenter, A.E.: Cell Profiler Analyst: data exploration and analysis software for complex image-based screens. BMC Bioinf. **9**(1), 482 (2008). https://doi.org/10.1186/1471-2105-9-482
276. Jönsson, D., Bergström, A., Forsell, C., Simon, R., Engström, M., Ynnerman, A., Hotz, I.: A visual environment for hypothesis formation and reasoning in studies with fMRI and multivariate clinical data. In: Proceeding of Eurographics Workshop on Visual Computing for Biology and Medicine, pp. 57–68 (2019). https://doi.org/10.2312/VCBM.20191232
277. Jönsson, D., Sundén, E., Ynnerman, A., Ropinski, T.: A survey of volumetric illumination techniques for interactive volume rendering. Comput. Graph. Forum **33**(1), 27–51 (2014). https://doi.org/10.1111/cgf.12252
278. Joshi, A., Qian, X., Dione, D., Bulsara, K., Breuer, C., Sinusas, A., Papademetris, X.: Effective visualization of complex vascular structures using a non-parametric vessel detection method. IEEE Trans. Vis. Comput. Graph. **14**(6), 1603–1610 (2008). https://doi.org/10.1109/tvcg.2008.123
279. Joshi, S.H., Bowman, I., Van Horn, J.D.: Large-scale neuroanatomical visualization using a manifold embedding approach. In: Proceeding of IEEE Symposium on Visual Analytics Science and Technology, pp. 237–238 (2010). https://doi.org/10.1109/tvcg.2008.123
280. Jung, Y., Kim, J., Bi, L., Kumar, A., Feng, D.D., Fulham, M.J.: A direct volume rendering visualization approach for serial PET-CT scans that preserves anatomical consistency. Int. J. Comput. Assist. Radiol. Surg. **14**(5), 733–744 (2019). https://doi.org/10.1007/s11548-019-01916-2
281. Jurčík, A., Parulek, J., Sochor, J., Kozlíková, B.: Accelerated visualization of transparent molecular surfaces in molecular dynamics. In: Proceeding of IEEE Pacific Visualization Symposium, pp. 112–119 (2016). https://doi.org/10.1109/pacificvis.2016.7465258

282. Kalia, M., Mathur, P., Tsang, K., Black, P., Navab, N., Salcudean, S.: Evaluation of a markerless, intra-operative, augmented reality guidance system for robot-assisted laparoscopic radical prostatectomy. Int. J. Comput. Assist. Radiol. Surg. **15**(7), 1225–1233 (2020). https://doi.org/10.1007/s11548-020-02181-4
283. Kammerer, S., Roth, R.B., Reneland, R., Marnellos, G., Hoyal, C.R., Markward, N.J., Ebner, F., et al.: Large-scale association study identifies ICAM gene region as breast and prostate cancer susceptibility locus. Can. Res. **64**(24), 8906–8910 (2004). https://doi.org/10.1158/0008-5472.can-04-1788
284. Kandalaft, M.R., Didehbani, N., Krawczyk, D.C., Allen, T.T., Chapman, S.B.: Virtual reality social cognition training for young adults with high-functioning autism. J. Autism Dev. Disord. **43**(1), 34–44 (2013). https://doi.org/10.1007/s10803-012-1544-6
285. Kanehisa, M.: KEGG: Kyoto encyclopedia of genes and genomes. Nucleic Acids Res. **28**(1), 27–30 (2000). https://doi.org/10.1093/nar/28.1.27
286. Kanitsar, A.: Curved planar reformation for vessel visualization. Ph.D. thesis, TU Wien (2004)
287. Kanitsar, A., Fleischmann, D., Wegenkittl, R., Felkel, P., Gröller, E.: CPR - curved planar reformation. In: Proceeding of IEEE Visualization (2002). https://doi.org/10.1109/visual.2002.1183754
288. Kanitsar, A., Wegenkittl, R., Fleischmann, D., Gröller, M.E.: Advanced curved planar reformation: Flattening of vascular structures. In: Proceeding of IEEE Visualization, pp. 43–50 (2003). https://doi.org/10.1109/visual.2003.1250353
289. Kanou, M., Nishimura, K., Hirota, K., Hirose, M., Aburatani, H., Hamakubo, T., Kodama, T.: Visualization for genome function analysis. In: Proceeding of IEEE Virtual Reality, pp. 301–302 (2001). https://doi.org/10.1109/VR.2001.913807
290. Kashani, Z.R.M., Ahrabian, H., Elahi, E., Nowzari-Dalini, A., Ansari, E.S., Asadi, S., Mohammadi, S., Schreiber, F., Masoudi-Nejad, A.: Kavosh: a new algorithm for finding network motifs. BMC Bioinf. **10**(1), 318 (2009). https://doi.org/10.1186/1471-2105-10-318
291. Kaufman, A., Wang, J.: 3D surface reconstruction from endoscopic videos. In: Visualization in Medicine and Life Sciences, pp. 61–74. Springer (2008). https://doi.org/10.1007/978-3-540-72630-24
292. Kaufman, A., Yagel, R., Bakalash, R., Spector, I.: Volume visualization in cell biology. In: Proceeding of IEEE Visualization, pp. 160–168 (1990)https://doi.org/10.1109/VISUAL.1990.146378
293. Keil, M., Laura, C.O., Drechsler, K., Wesarg, S.: Combining B-mode and color flow vessel segmentation for registration of hepatic CT and ultrasound volumes. In: Proceeding of Eurographics Workshop on Visual Computing in Biology and Medicine, pp. 57–64 (2012). https://doi.org/10.2312/VCBM/VCBM12/057-064
294. Kenoui, M., Mehdi, M.A.: Teach-Me DNA: an interactive course using voice output in an augmented reality system. In: Proceeding of Conference on Communications, Control Systems and Signal Processing, pp. 260–265 (2020). https://doi.org/10.1109/ccssp49278.2020.9151605
295. Kerbl, B., Kopanas, G., Leimkuehler, T., Drettakis, G.: 3D gaussian splatting for real-time radiance field rendering. ACM Trans. Graph. **42**(4) (2023). https://doi.org/10.1145/3592433
296. Kern, F., Winter, C., Gall, D., Käthner, I., Pauli, P., Latoschik, M.E.: Immersive virtual reality and gamification within procedurally generated environments to increase motivation during gait rehabilitation. In: Proceeding of IEEE Conference on Virtual Reality and 3D User Interfaces, pp. 500–509 (2019). https://doi.org/10.1109/vr.2019.8797828
297. Kersten-Oertel, M., Jannin, P., Collins, D.L.: DVV: a taxonomy for mixed reality visualization in image guided surgery. IEEE Trans. Vis. Comput. Graph. **18**(2), 332–352 (2011). https://doi.org/10.1109/TVCG.2011.50

298. Kikinis, R., Shenton, M.E., Iosifescu, D.V., McCarley, R.W., Saiviroonporn, P., Hokama, H.H., Robatino, A., Metcalf, D., Wible, C.G., Portas, C.M., et al.: A digital brain atlas for surgical planning, model-driven segmentation, and teaching. IEEE Trans. Vis. Comput. Graph. **2**(3), 232–241 (1996). https://doi.org/10.1109/2945.537306
299. Kim, K., Norouzi, N., Losekamp, T., Bruder, G., Anderson, M., Welch, G.: Effects of patient care assistant embodiment and computer mediation on user experience. In: Proceeding of IEEE Conference on Artificial Intelligence and Virtual Reality, pp. 17–177 (2019). https://doi.org/10.1109/aivr46125.2019.00013
300. Kim, N.W., Im, H., Henry Riche, N., Wang, A., Gajos, K., Pfister, H.: Dataselfie: Empowering people to design personalized visuals to represent their data. In: Proceeding of the CHI Conference on Human Factors in Computing Systems, pp. 1–12 (2019). https://doi.org/10.1145/3290605.3300309
301. Kindlmann, G.: Superquadric tensor glyphs. In: Proceeding of Eurographics-IEEE TCVG Conference on Visualization, pp. 147–154 (2004). https://doi.org/10.2312/VISSYM/VISSYM04/147-154
302. Kindlmann, G., Weinstein, D., Hart, D.: Strategies for direct volume rendering of diffusion tensor fields. IEEE Trans. Vis. Comput. Graph. **6**(2), 124–138 (2000). https://doi.org/10.1109/2945.856994
303. Klein, T., Autin, L., Kozlíková, B., Goodsell, D.S., Olson, A., Gröller, M.E., Viola, I.: Instant construction and visualization of crowded biological environments. IEEE Trans. Vis. Comput. Graph. **24**(1), 862–872 (2017). https://doi.org/10.1109/TVCG.2017.2744258
304. Klemm, P., Lawonn, K., Glaßer, S., Niemann, U., Hegenscheid, K., Völzke, H., Preim, B.: 3D regression heat map analysis of population study data. IEEE Trans. Vis. Comput. Graph. **22**(1), 81–90 (2016). https://doi.org/10.1109/TVCG.2015.2468291
305. Klemm, P., Oeltze-Jafra, S., Lawonn, K., Hegenscheid, K., Völzke, H., Preim, B.: Interactive visual analysis of image-centric cohort study data. IEEE Trans. Vis. Comput. Graph. **20**(12), 1673–1682 (2014). https://doi.org/10.1109/TVCG.2014.2346591
306. Kniss, J., Kindlmann, G., Hansen, C.: Multidimensional transfer functions for interactive volume rendering. IEEE Trans. Vis. Comput. Graph. **8**(3), 270–285 (2002). https://doi.org/10.1109/tvcg.2002.1021579
307. Kobak, D., Berens, P.: The art of using t-SNE for single-cell transcriptomics. Nat. Commun. **10**(1) (2019). https://doi.org/10.1038/s41467-019-13056-x
308. Kobak, D., Linderman, G.C.: Initialization is critical for preserving global data structure in both t-SNE and UMAP. Nat. Biotechnol. **39**(2), 156–157 (2021). https://doi.org/10.1038/s41587-020-00809-z
309. Kocev, B., Georgii, J., Linsen, L., Hahn, H.K.: Information fusion for real-time motion estimation in image-guided breast biopsy navigation. In: Proceeding of VRIPHYS, pp. 87–98 (2014). https://doi.org/10.2312/VRIPHYS.20141227
310. Kocincová, L., Jarešová, M., Byška, J., Parulek, J., Hauser, H., Kozlíková, B.: Comparative visualization of protein secondary structures. BMC Bioinformatics **18**(2), 1–12 (2017). https://doi.org/10.1186/S12859-016-1449-Z
311. Koepnick, S., Norpchen, D., Sherman, W.R., Coming, D.S.: Immersive training for two-person radiological surveys. In: Proceeding of IEEE Virtual Reality, pp. 171–174 (2009). https://doi.org/10.1109/vr.2009.4811018
312. Köhler, B., Gasteiger, R., Preim, U., Theisel, H., Gutberlet, M., Preim, B.: Semi-automatic vortex extraction in 4D PC-MRI cardiac blood flow data using line predicates. IEEE Trans. Vis. Comput. Graph. **19**(12), 2773–2782 (2013). https://doi.org/10.1109/tvcg.2013.189
313. Kohonen, T.: Self-organized formation of topologically correct feature maps. Biol. Cybern. **43**(1), 59–69 (1982). https://doi.org/10.1007/bf00337288

314. Kolesár, I., Byška, J., Parulek, J., Hauser, H., Kozlíková, B.: Unfolding and interactive exploration of protein tunnels and their dynamics. In: Proceeding of the Eurographics Workshop on Visual Computing for Biology and Medicine, pp. 1–10 (2016). https://doi.org/10.2312/VCBM.20161265
315. Kong, F., Wilson, N., Shadden, S.: A deep-learning approach for direct whole-heart mesh reconstruction. Med. Image Anal. **74**, 102222 (2021). https://doi.org/10.1016/j.media.2021.102222
316. Koradi, R., Billeter, M., Wüthrich, K.: MOLMOL: a program for display and analysis of macromolecular structures. J. Mol. Graph. **14**(1), 51–55 (1996). https://doi.org/10.1016/0263-7855(96)00009-4
317. Kottravel, S., Falk, M., Sundén, E., Ropinski, T.: Coverage-based opacity estimation for interactive depth of field in molecular visualization. In: Proceeding of IEEE Pacific Visualization Symposium, pp. 255–262 (2015). https://doi.org/10.1109/pacificvis.2015.7156385
318. Kouřil, D., Strnad, O., Mindek, P., Halladjian, S., Isenberg, T., Gröller, M.E., Viola, I.: Molecumentary: adaptable narrated documentaries using molecular visualization. IEEE Trans. Vis. Comput. Graph., 1733–1747 (2022). https://doi.org/10.1109/TVCG.2021.3130670
319. Koutek, M., van Hees, J., Post, F.H., Bakker, A.: Virtual spring manipulators for particle steering in molecular dynamics on the responsive workbench. In: Proceeding of the Eurographics Workshop on Virtual Environments, pp. 53–62 (2002). https://doi.org/10.2312/EGVE/EGVE02/053-062
320. Kozlíková, B., Krone, M., Falk, M., Lindow, N., Baaden, M., Baum, D., Viola, I., Parulek, J., Hege, H.C.: Visualization of biomolecular structures: state of the art revisited. Comput. Graph. Forum **36**(8), 178–204 (2017). https://doi.org/10.1111/CGF.13072
321. Kreiser, J., Meuschke, M., Mistelbauer, G., Preim, B., Ropinski, T.: A survey of flattening-based medical visualization techniques. Comput. Graph. Forum **37**(3), 597–624 (2018). https://doi.org/10.1111/CGF.13445
322. Kretschmer, J., Godenschwager, C., Preim, B., Stamminger, M.: Interactive patient-specific vascular modeling with sweep surfaces. IEEE Trans. Vis. Comput. Graph. **19**(12), 2828–2837 (2013). https://doi.org/10.1109/tvcg.2013.169
323. Kroes, T., Post, F.H., Botha, C.P.: Exposure render: an interactive photo-realistic volume rendering framework. PLoS ONE **7**(7), e38586 (2012). https://doi.org/10.1371/journal.pone.0038586
324. Krone, M., Grottel, S., Ertl, T.: Parallel contour-buildup algorithm for the molecular surface. In: Proceeding of IEEE Symposium on Biological Data Visualization, pp. 17–22 (2011). https://doi.org/10.1109/biovis.2011.6094043
325. Krone, M., Kozlíková, B., Lindow, N., Baaden, M., Baum, D., Parulek, J., Hege, H.C., Viola, I.: Visual analysis of biomolecular cavities: state of the art. Comput. Graph. Forum **35**(3), 527–551 (2016). https://doi.org/10.1111/cgf.12928
326. Krone, M., Reina, G., Schulz, C., Kulschewski, T., Pleiss, J., Ertl, T.: Interactive extraction and tracking of biomolecular surface features. Comput. Graph. Forum **32**(3), 331–340 (2013). https://doi.org/10.1111/CGF.12120
327. Krueger, R., Beyer, J., Jang, W.D., Kim, N.W., Sokolov, A., Sorger, P.K., Pfister, H.: Facetto: combining unsupervised and supervised learning for hierarchical phenotype analysis in multichannel image data. IEEE Trans. Vis. Comput. Graph. **26**(1), 227–237 (2019). https://doi.org/10.1109/TVCG.2019.2934547
328. Krüger, A., Kubisch, C., Strauß, G., Preim, B.: Advanced GPU volume rendering for virtual endoscopy. In: Proceeding of Eurographics—Medical Prize, pp. 13–16 (2009). https://doi.org/10.2312/EGM.20091026
329. Krüger, A., Tietjen, C., Hintze, J., Preim, B., Hertel, I., Strauß, G.: Interactive visualization for neck-dissection planning. In: Proceeding of EuroVis, pp. 295–302 (2005). https://doi.org/10.2312/VisSym/EuroVis05/295-302

330. Krzywinski, M., Schein, J., Birol, I., Connors, J., Gascoyne, R., Horsman, D., Jones, S.J., Marra, M.A.: Circos: an information aesthetic for comparative genomics. Genome Res. **19**(9), 1639–1645 (2009). https://doi.org/10.1101/gr.092759.109
331. Kubisch, C., Glaßer, S., Neugebauer, M., Preim, B.: Vessel visualization with volume rendering. In: Visualization in Medicine and Life Sciences II, pp. 109–132. Springer (2012). https://doi.org/10.1007/978-3-642-21608-47
332. Kubisch, C., Tietjen, C., Preim, B.: GPU-based smart visibility techniques for tumor surgery planning. Int. J. Comput. Assist. Radiol. Surg. **5**(6), 667–678 (2010). https://doi.org/10.1007/s11548-010-0420-0
333. Kuchroo, M., Huang, J., Wong, P., Grenier, J.C., Shung, D., Tong, A., Lucas, C., Klein, J., Burkhardt, D.B., Gigante, S., et al.: Multiscale PHATE identifies multimodal signatures of COVID-19. Nat. Biotechnol. **40**(5), 681–691 (2022). https://doi.org/10.1038/s41587-021-01186-x
334. Kultys, M., Nicholas, L., Schwarz, R., Goldman, N., King, J.: Sequence Bundles: a novel method for visualising, discovering and exploring sequence motifs. BMC Proc. **8**(2), S8 (2014). https://doi.org/10.1186/1753-6561-8-S2-S8
335. Kumamura, S., Niki, N., Nishitani, H., Sato, H.: 3D visualization of fuzzy shapes using multichannel MR images. In: Proceeding of IEEE Conference Record Nuclear Science Symposium and Medical Imaging Conference, pp. 1647–1651 (1993). https://doi.org/10.1109/nssmic.1993.373570
336. Kuntze, M.F., Stoermer, R., Mager, R., Roessler, A., Mueller-Spahn, F., Bullinger, A.H.: Immersive virtual environments in cue exposure. Cyberpsychol. Behav. **4**(4), 497–501 (2001). https://doi.org/10.1089/109493101750527051
337. Kurup, H.K., Samuel, B.P., Vettukattil, J.J.: Hybrid 3D printing: a game-changer in personalized cardiac medicine? Expert Rev. Cardiovasc. Ther. **13**(12), 1281–1284 (2015). https://doi.org/10.1586/14779072.2015.1100076
338. Kuß, A., Prohaska, S., Meyer, B., Rybak, J., Hege, H.C.: Ontology-based visualization of hierarchical neuroanatomical structures. In: Proceeding of Eurographics Workshop on Visual Computing in Biology and Medicine, pp. 177–184 (2008). https://doi.org/10.2312/VCBM/VCBM08/177-184
339. Kut̆ák, D., Selzer, M.N., Byška, J., Ganuza, M.L., Barisic, I., Kozlíková, B., Miao, H.: Vivern-a virtual environment for multiscale visualization and modeling of DNA nanostructures. IEEE Trans. Vis. Comput. Graph. **28**(12), 4825–4838 (2021). https://doi.org/10.1109/tvcg.2021.3106328
340. Kwon, B.C., Choi, M.J., Kim, J.T., Choi, E., Kim, Y.B., Kwon, S., Sun, J., Choo, J.: Retainvis: visual analytics with interpretable and interactive recurrent neural networks on electronic medical records. IEEE Trans. Vis. Comput. Graph. **25**(1), 299–309 (2018). https://doi.org/10.1109/tvcg.2018.2865027
341. Lacey, G., Ryan, D., Cassidy, D., Young, D.: Mixed-reality simulation of minimally invasive surgeries. IEEE Multimedia **14**(4), 76–87 (2007). https://doi.org/10.1109/mmul.2007.79
342. Laidlaw, D.H., Ahrens, E.T., Kremers, D., Avalos, M.J., Jacobs, R.E., Readhead, C.: Visualizing diffusion tensor images of the mouse spinal cord. In: Proceeding of IEEE Visualization, pp. 127–134 (1998). https://doi.org/10.1109/visual.1998.745294
343. Lam, H., Bertini, E., Isenberg, P., Plaisant, C., Carpendale, S.: Empirical studies in information visualization: seven scenarios. IEEE Trans. Vis. Comput. Graph. **18**(9), 1520–1536 (2011). https://doi.org/10.1109/TVCG.2011.279
344. Lambert, A., Dubois, J., Bourqui, R.: Pathway preserving representation of metabolic networks. Comput. Graph. Forum **30**(3), 1021–1030 (2011). https://doi.org/10.1111/j.1467-8659.2011.01951.x

345. Lander, E.S., Linton, L.M., Birren, B., Nusbaum, C., Zody, M.C., Baldwin, J., Devon, K., Dewar, K., Doyle, M., FitzHugh, W., Funke, R., et al.: Initial sequencing and analysis of the human genome. Nature **409**(6822), 860–921 (2001). https://doi.org/10.1038/35057062
346. Laskowski, R.A., Jabłońska, J., Pravda, L., Vařeková, R.S., Thornton, J.M.: PDBsum: structural summaries of PDB entries. Protein Sci. **27**(1), 129–134 (2018). https://doi.org/10.1002/pro.3289
347. Laskowski, R.A., Swindells, M.B.: LigPlot+: multiple ligand-protein interaction diagrams for drug discovery. J. Chem. Inf. Model. **51**(10), 2778–2786 (2011). https://doi.org/10.1021/CI200227U
348. Läthén, G., Lindholm, S., Lenz, R., Persson, A., Borga, M.: Automatic tuning of spatially varying transfer functions for blood vessel visualization. IEEE Trans. Vis. Comput. Graph. **18**(12), 2345–2354 (2012). https://doi.org/10.1109/tvcg.2012.203
349. Lawonn, K., Gasteiger, R., Preim, B.: Adaptive surface visualization of vessels with animated blood flow. Comput. Graph. Forum **33**(8), 16–27 (2014). https://doi.org/10.1111/CGF.12355
350. Lawonn, K., Glaßer, S., Vilanova, A., Preim, B., Isenberg, T.: Occlusion-free blood flow animation with wall thickness visualization. IEEE Trans. Vis. Comput. Graph. **22**(1), 728–737 (2015). https://doi.org/10.1109/TVCG.2015.2467961
351. Lawonn, K., Krone, M., Ertl, T., Preim, B.: Line integral convolution for real-time illustration of molecular surface shape and salient regions. Comput. Graph. Forum **33**(3), 181–190 (2014). https://doi.org/10.1111/CGF.12374
352. Lawonn, K., Luz, M., Preim, B., Hansen, C.: Illustrative visualization of vascular models for static 2D representations. In: Proceeding of Medical Image Computing and Computer-Assisted Intervention, pp. 399–406 (2015). https://doi.org/10.1007/978-3-319-24571-348
353. Lawonn, K., Mönch, T., Preim, B.: Streamlines for illustrative real-time rendering. Comput. Graph. Forum **32**(3), 321–330 (2013). https://doi.org/10.1111/CGF.12119
354. Lawonn, K., Preim, B.: Feature lines for illustrating medical surface models: Mathematical background and survey. In: Visualization in Medicine and Life Sciences III, pp. 93–131. Springer (2016). https://doi.org/10.1007/978-3-319-24523-25
355. Lawonn, K., Smit, N.N., Bühler, K., Preim, B.: A survey on multimodal medical data visualization. Comput. Graph. Forum **37**(1), 413–438 (2018). https://doi.org/10.1111/CGF.13306
356. Lawonn, K., Viola, I., Preim, B., Isenberg, T.: A survey of surface-based illustrative rendering for visualization. Comput. Graph. Forum **37**(6), 205–234 (2018). https://doi.org/10.1111/cgf.13322
357. Lawrence, M., Lee, E.K., Cook, D., Hofmann, H., Wurtele, E.: exploRase: Exploratory Data Analysis of Systems Biology Data. In: Proceeding of International Conference on Coordinated & Multiple Views in Exploratory Visualization (CMV (2006). https://doi.org/10.1109/cmv.2006.7
358. Le Muzic, M., Autin, L., Parulek, J., Viola, I.: cellVIEW: a tool for illustrative and multi-scale rendering of large biomolecular datasets. In: Proceeding of Eurographics Workshop on Visual Computing for Biomedicine, vol. 2015, pp. 61–70 (2015). https://doi.org/10.2312/VCBM.20151209
359. Le Muzic, M., Parulek, J., Stavrum, A.K., Viola, I.: Illustrative visualization of molecular reactions using omniscient intelligence and passive agents. Comput. Graph. Forum **33**(3), 141–150 (2014). https://doi.org/10.1111/CGF.12370
360. Lee, B., Richards, F.M.: The interpretation of protein structures: estimation of static accessibility. J. Mol. Biol. **55**(3), 379–IN4 (1971). https://doi.org/10.1016/0022-2836(71)90324-x
361. Lee, C.H., Varshney, A.: Computing and displaying intermolecular negative volume for docking. In: Scientific Visualization: The Visual Extraction of Knowledge from Data, pp. 49–64. Springer (2006). https://doi.org/10.1007/3-540-30790-74

362. Leith, A., Marko, M., Parsons, D.: Computer graphics for cellular reconstruction. IEEE Comput. Graph. Appl. **9**(05), 16–23 (1989). https://doi.org/10.1109/38.35534
363. Leung, C.K., Chen, Y., Hoi, C.S., Shang, S., Wen, Y., Cuzzocrea, A.: Big data visualization and visual analytics of COVID-19 data. In: Proceeding of Information Visualisation, pp. 415–420 (2020). https://doi.org/10.1109/iv51561.2020.00073
364. Levine, D., Facello, M., Hallstrom, P., Reeder, G., Walenz, B., Stevens, F.: Stalk: an interactive system for virtual molecular docking. IEEE Comput. Sci. Eng. **4**(2), 55–65 (1997). https://doi.org/10.1109/99.609834
365. Levine, J.H., Simonds, E.F., Bendall, S.C., Davis, K.L., ad D. Amir, E., Tadmor, M.D., Litvin, O., Fienberg, H.G., Jager, A., Zunder, E.R., Finck, R., Gedman, A.L., Radtke, I., Downing, J.R., Pe'er, D., Nolan, G.P.: Data-driven phenotypic dissection of AML reveals progenitor-like cells that correlate with prognosis. Cell **162**(1), 184–197 (2015). https://doi.org/10.1016/j.cell.2015.05.047
366. Levoy, M.: Efficient ray tracing of volume data. ACM Trans. Graph. **9**(3), 245–261 (1990). https://doi.org/10.1145/78964.78965
367. Levoy, M., Fuchs, H., Pizer, S.M., Rosenman, J., Chaney, E.L., Sherouse, G.W., Interrante, V., Kiel, J.: Volume rendering in radiation treatment planning. In: Proceeding of Visualization in Biomedical Computing, pp. 4–10 (1990). https://doi.org/10.1109/vbc.1990.109295
368. Lex, A., Gehlenborg, N., Strobelt, H., Vuillemot, R., Pfister, H.: UpSet: visualization of intersecting sets. IEEE Trans. Vis. Comput. Graph. **20**(12), 1983–1992 (2014). https://doi.org/10.1109/TVCG.2014.2346248
369. Li, S., Wakefield, J., Noble, J.A.: Automated segmentation and alignment of mitotic nuclei for kymograph visualisation. In: Proceeding of IEEE International Symposium on Biomedical Imaging: From Nano to Macro, pp. 622–625 (2011). https://doi.org/10.1109/isbi.2011.5872484
370. Li, W., Kaufman, A., Kreeger, K.: Real-time volume rendering for virtual colonoscopy. In: Proceeding of Volume Graphics, pp. 363–374 (2001). https://doi.org/10.1007/978-3-7091-6756-425
371. Liang, Z., Ploderer, B., Liu, W., Nagata, Y., Bailey, J., Kulik, L., Li, Y.: SleepExplorer: a visualization tool to make sense of correlations between personal sleep data and contextual factors. Pers. Ubiquit. Comput. **20**(6), 985–1000 (2016). https://doi.org/10.1007/s00779-016-0960-6
372. Liao, H., Inomata, T., Sakuma, I., Dohi, T.: 3-D augmented reality for MRI-guided surgery using integral videography autostereoscopic image overlay. IEEE Trans. Biomed. Eng. **57**(6), 1476–1486 (2010). https://doi.org/10.1109/tbme.2010.2040278
373. Lichtenberg, N., Smit, N.N., Hansen, C., Lawonn, K.: Sline: Seamless line illustration for interactive biomedical visualization. In: Proceeding of Eurographics Workshop on Visual Computing for Biology and Medicine, pp. 133–142 (2016). https://doi.org/10.5555/3061507.3061529
374. Lindemann, F., Laukamp, K., Jacobs, A.H., Hinrichs, K.H.: Interactive comparative visualization of multimodal brain tumor segmentation data. In: Proceeding of Vision, Modeling & Visualization, pp. 105–112 (2013). https://doi.org/10.2312/PE.VMV.VMV13.105-112
375. Linderman, G.C., Rachh, M., Hoskins, J.G., Steinerberger, S., Kluger, Y.: Fast interpolation-based t-SNE for improved visualization of single-cell RNA-seq data. Nat. Methods **16**(3), 243–245 (2019). https://doi.org/10.1038/s41592-018-0308-4
376. Lindner, P., Rozental, A., Jurell, A., Reuterskiöld, L., Andersson, G., Hamilton, W., Miloff, A., Carlbring, P.: Experiences of gamified and automated virtual reality exposure therapy for spider phobia: Qualitative study. JMIR Serious Game. **8**(2), e17807 (2020). https://doi.org/10.2196/17807
377. Lindow, N., Baum, D., Bondar, A.N., Hege, H.C.: Exploring cavity dynamics in biomolecular systems. BMC Bioinformatics **14**(Suppl 19), S5 (2013). https://doi.org/10.1186/1471-2105-14-S19-S5

378. Lindow, N., Baum, D., Hege, H.C.: Ligand excluded surface: a new type of molecular surface. IEEE Trans. Vis. Comput. Graph. **20**(12), 2486–2495 (2014). https://doi.org/10.1109/tvcg.2014.2346404
379. Lindow, N., Baum, D., Prohaska, S., Hege, H.C.: Accelerated visualization of dynamic molecular surfaces. Comput. Graph. Forum **29**(3), 943–952 (2010). https://doi.org/10.1111/J.1467-8659.2009.01693.X
380. Linsen, L., Al-Taie, A., Ristovski, G., Preusser, T., Hahn, H.K.: Uncertainty and reproducibility in medical visualization. In: Proceeding of EuroVis Workshop on Reproducibility, Verification, and Validation in Visualization, pp. 1–3 (2016). https://doi.org/10.2312/eurorv3.20161107
381. Liu, P., Liu, S., Fang, Y., Xue, X., Zou, J., Tseng, G., Konnikova, L.: Recent advances in computer-assisted algorithms for cell subtype identification of cytometry data. Front. Cell Dev. Biol. **8** (2020). https://doi.org/10.3389/fcell.2020.00234
382. Ljung, P., Krüger, J., Gröller, E., Hadwiger, M., Hansen, C.D., Ynnerman, A.: State of the art in transfer functions for direct volume rendering. Comput. Graph. Forum **35**(3), 669–691 (2016). https://doi.org/10.1111/cgf.12934
383. Ljung, P., Lundstrom, C., Ynnerman, A., Museth, K.: Transfer function based adaptive decompression for volume rendering of large medical data sets. In: Proceeding of IEEE Symposium on Volume Visualization and Graphics, pp. 25–32 (2004). https://doi.org/10.1109/SVVG.2004.14
384. Long, T.V., Linsen, L.: Supervised kernel principal component analysis for visual sample-based analysis of gene expression data. In: Visualization in Medicine and Life Sciences (2013). https://doi.org/10.2312/PE.VMLS.VMLS2013.055-059
385. Lorensen, W.E., Cline, H.E.: Marching Cubes: a high resolution 3D surface construction algorithm. In: ACM SIGGRAPH Computer Graphics, vol. 21(4), pp. 163–169 (1987). https://doi.org/10.1145/37402.37422
386. Lozano, J.A., Montesa, J., Juan, M.C., Alcañiz, M., Rey, B., Gil, J., Martinez, J.M., Gaggioli, A., Morganti, F.: VR-Mirror: a virtual reality system for mental practice in post-stroke rehabilitation. In: Proceeding of Smart Graphics, pp. 241–251 (2005). https://doi.org/10.1007/1153648223
387. Lundstrom, C., Rydell, T., Forsell, C., Persson, A., Ynnerman, A.: Multi-touch table system for medical visualization: application to orthopedic surgery planning. IEEE Trans. Vis. Comput. Graph. **17**(12), 1775–1784 (2011). https://doi.org/10.1109/tvcg.2011.224
388. Lv, Z., Tek, A., Da Silva, F., Empereur-Mot, C., Chavent, M., Baaden, M.: Game on, science-how video game technology may help biologists tackle visualization challenges. PLoS ONE **8**(3), e57990 (2013). https://doi.org/10.1371/journal.pone.0057990
389. Maas, K.W.H., Pezzotti, N., Vermeer, A.J.E., Ruijters, D., Vilanova, A.: NeRF for 3D reconstruction from X-ray angiography: possibilities and limitations. In: Eurographics Workshop on Visual Computing for Biology and Medicine (2023). https://doi.org/10.2312/vcbm.20231210
390. van der Maaten, L., Hinton, G.: Visualizing data using t-SNE. J. Mach. Learn. Res. **9**(86), 2579–2605 (2008)
391. Maciejewski, R., Livengood, P., Rudolph, S., Collins, T.F., Ebert, D.S., Brigantic, R.T., Corley, C.D., Muller, G.A., Sanders, S.W.: A pandemic influenza modeling and visualization tool. J. Vis. Lang. Comput. **22**(4), 268–78 (2011). https://doi.org/10.1016/j.jvlc.2011.04.002
392. Maciejewski, R., Rudolph, S., Hafen, R., Abusalah, A.M., Yakout, M., Ouzzani, M., Cleveland, W.S., Grannis, S.J., Wade, M., Ebert, D.S.: Understanding syndromic hotspots—a visual analytics approach. In: Proceeding of IEEE Symposium on Visual Analytics Science and Technology, pp. 35–42 (2008). https://doi.org/10.1109/vast.2008.4677354
393. Maduranga, U., Wijegunarathna, K., Weerasinghe, S., Perera, I., Wickramarachchi, A.: Dimensionality reduction for cluster identification in metagenomics using autoencoders. In: Proceed-

ing of International Conference on Advances in ICT for Emerging Regions (2020). https://doi.org/10.1109/icter51097.2020.9325447

394. Martschinke, J., Hartnagel, S., Keinert, B., Engel, K., Stamminger, M.: Adaptive temporal sampling for volumetric path tracing of medical data. Comput. Graph. Forum **38**(4), 67–76 (2019). https://doi.org/10.1111/cgf.13771
395. Martschinke, J., Klein, V., Kurth, P., Engel, K., Ludolph, I., Hauck, T., Horch, R., Stamminger, M.: Projection mapping for in-situ surgery planning by the example of DIEP flap breast reconstruction. In: Proceeding of Eurographics Workshop on Visual Computing for Biology and Medicine (2021). https://doi.org/10.2312/vcbm.20211354
396. Massie, T.H., Salisbury, J.K.: The phantom haptic interface: A device for probing virtual objects. In: Proceeding of the ASME Winter Annual Meeting, Symposium on Haptic Interfaces for Virtual Environment and Teleoperator Systems, vol. 55-1, pp. 295–300 (1994)
397. Masutani, Y., Masamune, K., Dohi, T.: Region-growing based feature extraction algorithm for tree-like objects. In: Proceeding of Visualization in Biomedical Computing, pp. 159–171 (1996). https://doi.org/10.1007/bfb0046951
398. Max, N.: Computer representation of molecular surfaces. IEEE Comput. Graph. Appl. **3**(05), 21–29 (1983). https://doi.org/10.1109/mcg.1983.263183
399. Mayoral, R., Tsagarakis, N., Petrone, M., Clapworthy, G., Caldwell, D., Zannoni, C.: Integration of haptic and visual modalities for a total hip replacement planning system. In: Proceeding of Medical Information Visualisation–Biomedical Visualisation, pp. 30–35 (2005). https://doi.org/10.1109/medivis.2005.11
400. McInnes, L., Healy, J., Melville, J.: UMAP: uniform manifold approximation and projection for dimension reduction (2018). https://doi.org/10.48550/ARXIV.1802.03426
401. Meißner, M., Huang, J., Bartz, D., Mueller, K., Crawfis, R.: A practical evaluation of popular volume rendering algorithms. In: Proceeding of IEEE Symposium on Volume Visualization, pp. 81–90 (2000). https://doi.org/10.1145/353888.353903
402. Meuschke, M., Garrison, L.A., Smit, N.N., Bach, B., Mittenentzwei, S., Weiß, V., Bruckner, S., Lawonn, K., Preim, B.: Narrative medical visualization to communicate disease data. Comput. Graph. **107**, 144–157 (2022). https://doi.org/10.1016/j.cag.2022.07.017
403. Meuschke, M., Günther, T., Wickenhöfer, R., Gross, M., Preim, B., Lawonn, K.: Management of cerebral aneurysm descriptors based on an automatic ostium extraction. IEEE Comput. Graph. Appl. **38**(3), 58–72 (2018). https://doi.org/10.1109/mcg.2018.032421654
404. Meuschke, M., Köhler, B., Preim, U., Preim, B., Lawonn, K.: Semi-automatic vortex flow classification in 4D PC-MRI data of the aorta. Comput. Graph. Forum **35**(3), 351–360 (2016). https://doi.org/10.1111/CGF.12911
405. Meuschke, M., Niemann, U., Behrendt, B., Gutberlet, M., Preim, B., Lawonn, K.: GUCCI–guided cardiac cohort investigation of blood flow data. IEEE Trans. Vis. Comput. Graph. **29**(3), 1876–1892 (2023). https://doi.org/10.1109/TVCG.2021.3134083
406. Meyer, M., Munzner, T., DePace, A., Pfister, H.: MulteeSum: a tool for comparative spatial and temporal gene expression data. IEEE Trans. Vis. Comput. Graph. **16**(6), 908–917 (2010). https://doi.org/10.1109/tvcg.2010.137
407. Meyer, M., Munzner, T., Pfister, H.: MizBee: a multiscale synteny browser. IEEE Trans. Vis. Comput. Graph. **15**(6), 897–904 (2009). https://doi.org/10.1109/tvcg.2009.167
408. Meyer-Spradow, J., Ropinski, T., Hinrichs, K.: Supporting depth and motion perception in medical volume data. In: Visualization in Medicine and Life Sciences, pp. 121–133 (2008). https://doi.org/10.1007/978-3-540-72630-27
409. Miao, H., Klein, T., Kouřil, D., Mindek, P., Schatz, K., Gröller, M.E., Kozlíková, B., Isenberg, T., Viola, I.: Multiscale molecular visualization. J. Mol. Biol. **431**(6), 1049–1070 (2019). https://doi.org/10.1016/j.jmb.2018.09.004

410. Miao, H., Mistelbauer, G., Karimov, A., Alansary, A., Davidson, A., Lloyd, D.F.A., Damodaram, M., Story, L., Hutter, J., Hajnal, J.V., Rutherford, M., Preim, B., Kainz, B., Gröller, M.E.: Placenta maps: in utero placental health assessment of the human fetus. IEEE Trans. Vis. Comput. Graph. **23**(6), 1612–1623 (2017). https://doi.org/10.1109/tvcg.2017.2674938
411. Miao, H., Mistelbauer, G., Našel, C., Gröller, M.E.: Visual quantification of the Circle of Willis: An automated identification and standardized representation. Comput. Graph. Forum **36**(6), 393–404 (2017). https://doi.org/10.1111/CGF.12988
412. Mildenhall, B., Srinivasan, P.P., Tancik, M., Barron, J.T., Ramamoorthi, R., Ng, R.: NeRF: representing scenes as neural radiance fields for view synthesis. Commun. ACM **65**(1), 99–106 (2021). https://doi.org/10.1145/3503250
413. Mirhosseini, S., Gutenko, I., Ojal, S., Marino, J., Kaufman, A.: Immersive virtual colonoscopy. IEEE Trans. Vis. Comput. Graph. **25**(5), 2011–2021 (2019). https://doi.org/10.1109/tvcg.2019.2898763
414. Mistelbauer, G., Morar, A., Varchola, A., Schernthaner, R., Baclija, I., Köchl, A., Kanitsar, A., Bruckner, S., Gröller, M.E.: Vessel visualization using curvicircular feature aggregation. Comput. Graph. Forum **32**(3), 231–240 (2013). https://doi.org/10.1111/CGF.12110
415. Mistelbauer, G., Rössl, C., Bäumler, K., Preim, B., Fleischmann, D.: Implicit modeling of patient-specific aortic dissections with elliptic fourier descriptors. Comput. Graph. Forum **40**(3), 423–434 (2021). https://doi.org/10.1111/CGF.14318
416. Mittenentzwei, S., Weiß, V., Schreiber, S., Garrison, L.A., Bruckner, S., Pfister, M., Preim, B., Meuschke, M.: Do disease stories need a hero? effects of human protagonists on a narrative visualization about cerebral small vessel disease. Comput. Graph. Forum **42**(3), 123–135 (2023). https://doi.org/10.1111/CGF.14817
417. Moench, T., Adler, S., Preim, B.: Staircase-aware smoothing of medical surface meshes. In: Proceeding of Eurographics Workshop on Visual Computing for Biology and Medicine, pp. 83–90 (2010). https://doi.org/10.2312/VCBM/VCBM10/083-090
418. Moench, T., Gasteiger, R., Janiga, G., Theisel, H., Preim, B.: Context-aware mesh smoothing for biomedical applications. Comput. Graph. **35**(4), 755–767 (2011). https://doi.org/10.1016/j.cag.2011.04.011
419. Mohammed, H., Al-Awami, A.K., Beyer, J., Cali, C., Magistretti, P., Pfister, H., Hadwiger, M.: Abstractocyte: a visual tool for exploring nanoscale astroglial cells. IEEE Trans. Vis. Comput. Graph. **24**(1), 853–861 (2017). https://doi.org/10.1109/TVCG.2017.2744278
420. Mönch, J., Mühler, K., Hansen, C., Oldhafer, K.J., Stavrou, G., Hillert, C., Logge, C., Preim, B.: The LiverSurgeryTrainer: training of computer-based planning in liver resection surgery. Int. J. Comput. Assist. Radiol. Surg. **8**(5), 809–818 (2013). https://doi.org/10.1007/S11548-013-0812-Z
421. Mönch, T., Lawonn, K., Kubisch, C., Westermann, R., Preim, B.: Interactive mesh smoothing for medical applications. Comput. Graph. Forum **32**(8), 110–121 (2013). https://doi.org/10.1111/cgf.12165
422. Monroe, M., Lan, R., Lee, H., Plaisant, C., Shneiderman, B.: Temporal event sequence simplification. IEEE Trans. Vis. Comput. Graph. **19**(12), 2227–2236 (2013). https://doi.org/10.1109/tvcg.2013.200
423. Montgomery, K., Bruyns, C., Wildermuth, S.: A virtual environment for simulated rat dissection: a case study of visualization for astronaut training. In: Proceeding of IEEE Visualization, pp. 509–601 (2001). https://doi.org/10.1109/visual.2001.964564
424. Moon, K.R., van Dijk, D., Wang, Z., Gigante, S., Burkhardt, D.B., Chen, W.S., Yim, K., van den Elzen, A., Hirn, M.J., Coifman, R.R., Ivanova, N.B., Wolf, G., Krishnaswamy, S.: Visualizing structure and transitions in high-dimensional biological data. Nat. Biotechnol. **37**(12), 1482–1492 (2019). https://doi.org/10.1038/s41587-019-0336-3

425. Mörth, E., Haldorsen, I.S., Bruckner, S., Smit, N.N.: ParaGlyder: probe-driven interactive visual analysis for multiparametric medical imaging data. In: Advances in Computer Graphics, pp. 351–363 (2020). https://doi.org/10.1007/978-3-030-61864-329
426. Mörth, E., Wagner-Larsen, K., Hodneland, E., Krakstad, C., Haldorsen, I.S., Bruckner, S., Smit, N.N.: RadEx: integrated visual exploration of multiparametric studies for radiomic tumor profiling. Comput. Graph. Forum **39**(7), 611–622 (2020). https://doi.org/10.1111/CGF.14172
427. Mosegaard, J., Sorensen, T.S.: GPU accelerated surgical simulators for complex morphology. In: Proceeding of IEEE Virtual Reality, pp. 147–153 (2005). https://doi.org/10.1109/vr.2005.1492768
428. Mühler, K., Preim, B.: Reusable visualizations and animations for surgery planning. Comput. Graph. Forum **29**(3), 1103–1112 (2010). https://doi.org/10.1111/J.1467-8659.2009.01669.X
429. Müller, J., Stoehr, M., Oeser, A., Gaebel, J., Streit, M., Dietz, A., Oeltze-Jafra, S.: A visual approach to explainable computerized clinical decision support. Comput. Graph. **91**, 1–11 (2020). https://doi.org/10.1016/j.cag.2020.06.004
430. Murray, P., McGee, F., Forbes, A.G.: A taxonomy of visualization tasks for the analysis of biological pathway data. BMC Bioinformatics **18**(S2), 21 (2017). https://doi.org/10.1186/s12859-016-1443-5
431. Neugebauer, M., Gasteiger, R., Beuing, O., Diehl, V., Skalej, M., Preim, B.: Map displays for the analysis of scalar data on cerebral aneurysm surfaces. Comput. Graph. Forum **28**(3), 895–902 (2009). https://doi.org/10.1111/J.1467-8659.2009.01459.X
432. Neugebauer, M., Janiga, G., Beuing, O., Skalej, M., Preim, B.: Anatomy-guided multi-level exploration of blood flow in cerebral aneurysms. Comput. Graph. Forum **30**(3), 1041–1050 (2011). https://doi.org/10.1111/J.1467-8659.2011.01953.X
433. Neugebauer, M., Lawonn, K., Beuing, O., Berg, P., Janiga, G., Preim, B.: AmniVis-A system for qualitative exploration of near-wall hemodynamics in cerebral aneurysms. Comput. Graph. Forum **32**(3), 251–260 (2013). https://doi.org/10.1111/CGF.12112
434. New, J., Kendall, W., Huang, J., Chesler, E.: Dynamic visualization of coexpression in systems genetics data. IEEE Trans. Vis. Comput. Graph. **14**(5), 1081–1095 (2008). https://doi.org/10.1109/tvcg.2008.61
435. Ney, D.R., Fishman, E.K., Magid, D., Drebin, R.A.: Volumetric rendering of computed tomography data: principles and techniques. IEEE Comput. Graph. Appl. **10**(2), 24–32 (1990). https://doi.org/10.1109/38.50670
436. Nguyen, B.P., Tay, W.L., Chui, C.K., Ong, S.H.: A clustering-based system to automate transfer function design for medical image visualization. Vis. Comput. **28**(2), 181–191 (2011). https://doi.org/10.1007/s00371-011-0634-3
437. Nguyen, Q.V., Huang, M.L., Qian, Y., Zhang, K.: A technique for visualizing dihedral signal of large protein sequences. In: Proceeding of Computer Graphics, Imaging and Visualisation, pp. 6–11 (2006). https://doi.org/10.1109/CGIV.2006.12
438. Nguyen, T., Plishker, W., Matisoff, A., Sharma, K., Shekhar, R.: HoloUS: augmented reality visualization of live ultrasound images using hololens for ultrasound-guided procedures. Int. J. Comput. Assist. Radiol. Surg. **17**(2), 385–391 (2022). https://doi.org/10.1007/s11548-021-02526-7
439. Nielsen, C.B., Cantor, M., Dubchak, I., Gordon, D., Wang, T.: Visualizing genomes: techniques and challenges. Nat. Methods **7**(3), S5–S15 (2010). https://doi.org/10.1038/nmeth.1422
440. Nielsen, C.B., Jackman, S.D., Birol, I., Jones, S.J.: ABySS-Explorer: visualizing genome sequence assemblies. IEEE Trans. Vis. Comput. Graph. **15**(6), 881–888 (2009). https://doi.org/10.1109/TVCG.2009.116
441. Nir-Hadad, S.Y., Weiss, P.L., Waizman, A., Schwartz, N., Kizony, R.: A virtual shopping task for the assessment of executive functions: validity for people with stroke. Neuropsychol. Rehabil. **27**(5), 808–833 (2017). https://doi.org/10.1080/09602011.2015.1109523

442. Nissler, C., Nowak, M., Connan, M., Büttner, S., Vogel, J., Kossyk, I., Márton, Z.C., Castellini, C.: VITA-an everyday virtual reality setup for prosthetics and upper-limb rehabilitation. J. Neural Eng. **16**(2), 026039 (2019). https://doi.org/10.1088/1741-2552/aaf35f
443. Noizet, M., Peltier, V., Deleau, H., Dauchez, M., Prévost, S., Jonquet-Prevoteau, J.: A collaborative molecular graphics tool for knowledge dissemination with augmented reality and 3D printing. In: Proceeding of Workshop on Molecular Graphics and Visual Analysis of Molecular Data, pp. 1–5 (2021). https://doi.org/10.2312/MOLVA.20211071
444. North, M.M., North, S.M., Coble, J.R.: Effectiveness of virtual environment desensitization in the treatment of agoraphobia. Presence Teleoper. Virtual Environ. **5**(3), 346–352 (1996). https://doi.org/10.1162/pres.1996.5.3.346
445. Nunes, M., Rowland, B., Schlachter, M., Ken, S., Matkovic, K., Laprie, A., Bühler, K.: An integrated visual analysis system for fusing MR spectroscopy and multi-modal radiology imaging. In: Proceeding of IEEE Symposium on Visual Analytics Science and Technology, pp. 53–62 (2014). https://doi.org/10.1109/vast.2014.7042481
446. Nusrat, S., Harbig, T., Gehlenborg, N.: Tasks, techniques, and tools for genomic data visualization. Comput. Graph. Forum **38**(3), 781–805 (2019). https://doi.org/10.1111/cgf.13727
447. O'Brien, T., Ritz, A., Raphael, B., Laidlaw, D.: Gremlin: an interactive visualization model for analyzing genomic rearrangements. IEEE Trans. Vis. Comput. Graph. **16**(6), 918–926 (2010). https://doi.org/10.1109/TVCG.2010.163
448. O'Donoghue, S.I.: Grand challenges in bioinformatics data visualization. Front. Bioinf. **1**, 669186 (2021). https://doi.org/10.3389/fbinf.2021.669186
449. O'Donoghue, S.I., Sabir, K.S., Kalemanov, M., Stolte, C., Wellmann, B., Ho, V., Roos, M., Perdigão, N., Buske, F.A., Heinrich, J., et al.: Aquaria: simplifying discovery and insight from protein structures. Nat. Methods **12**(2), 98–99 (2015). https://doi.org/10.1038/nmeth.3258
450. Oeltze, S., Doleisch, H., Hauser, H., Muigg, P., Preim, B.: Interactive visual analysis of perfusion data. IEEE Trans. Vis. Comput. Graph. **13**(6), 1392–1399 (2007). https://doi.org/10.1109/tvcg.2007.70569
451. Oeltze, S., Preim, B.: Visualization of anatomic tree structures with convolution surfaces. In: Proceeding of VisSym, pp. 311–320 (2004). https://doi.org/10.2312/VISSYM/VISSYM04/311-320
452. Oeltze-Jafra, S., Preim, B.: Survey of labeling techniques in medical visualizations. In: Proceeding of Eurographics Workshop on Visual Computing for Biology and Medicine, pp. 199–208 (2014). https://doi.org/10.2312/vcbm.20141192
453. Ohtake, Y., Belyaev, A.G., Alexa, M., Turk, G., Seidel, H.: Multi-level partition of unity implicits. ACM Trans. Graph. **22**(3), 463–470 (2003). https://doi.org/10.1145/882262.882293
454. Ola, O., Sedig, K.: The challenge of big data in public health: an opportunity for visual analytics. Online J. Public Health Inf. **5**(3), 223 (2014). https://doi.org/10.5210/ojphi.v5i3.4933
455. Olofsson, I., Lundin, K., Cooper, M., Kjall, P., Ynnerman, A.: A haptic interface for dose planning in stereo-tactic radiosurgery. In: Proceeding of Information Visualisation, pp. 200–205 (2004). https://doi.org/10.1109/iv.2004.5
456. Ornatsky, O.I., Kinach, R., Bandura, D.R., Lou, X., Tanner, S.D., Baranov, V.I., Nitz, M., Winnik, M.A.: Development of analytical methods for multiplex bio-assay with inductively coupled plasma mass spectrometry. J. Anal. At. Spectrom. **23**(4), 463 (2008). https://doi.org/10.1039/b710510j
457. Ostler, D., Seibold, M., Fuchtmann, J., Samm, N., Feussner, H., Wilhelm, D., Navab, N.: Acoustic signal analysis of instrument-tissue interaction for minimally invasive interventions. Int. J. Comput. Assist. Radiol. Surg. **15**(5), 771–779 (2020). https://doi.org/10.1007/s11548-020-02146-7
458. Otten, R., Vilanova, A., Van De Wetering, H.: Illustrative white matter fiber bundles. Comput. Graph. Forum **29**(3), 1013–1022 (2010). https://doi.org/10.1111/J.1467-8659.2009.01688.X

459. Owczarczyk, J., Owczarczyk, B.: Evaluation of true 3D display systems for visualizing medical volume data. Vis. Comput. **6**, 219–226 (2006). https://doi.org/10.1007/BF02341046
460. Pálenik, J., Byška, J., Bruckner, S., Hauser, H.: Scale-space splatting: reforming spacetime for cross-scale exploration of integral measures in molecular dynamics. IEEE Trans. Vis. Comput. Graph. **26**(1), 643–653 (2019). https://doi.org/10.1109/tvcg.2019.2934258
461. Palomar, R., Cheikh, F.A., Edwin, B., Beghdadhi, A., Elle, O.J.: Surface reconstruction for planning and navigation of liver resections. Comput. Med. Imaging Graph. **53**, 30–42 (2016). https://doi.org/10.1016/j.compmedimag.2016.07.003
462. Pankau, T., Wichmann, G., Neumuth, T., Preim, B., Dietz, A., Stumpp, P., Boehm, A.: 3D model-based documentation with the tumor therapy manager (TTM) improves TNM staging of head and neck tumor patients. Int. J. Comput. Assist. Radiol. Surg. **10**(10), 1617–1624 (2015). https://doi.org/10.1007/s11548-014-1131-8
463. Park, J.W., Nahm, F.S., Kim, J.H., Jeon, Y.T., Ryu, J.H., Han, S.H.: The effect of mirroring display of virtual reality tour of the operating theatre on preoperative anxiety: a randomized controlled trial. IEEE J. Biomed. Health Inform. **23**(6), 2655–2660 (2019). https://doi.org/10.1109/jbhi.2019.2892485
464. Parks, D.R., Roederer, M., Moore, W.A.: A new logicle display method avoids deceptive effects of logarithmic scaling for low signals and compensated data. Cytometry A **69A**(6), 541–551 (2006). https://doi.org/10.1002/cyto.a.20258
465. Partl, C., Lex, A., Streit, M., Kalkofen, D., Kashofer, K., Schmalstieg, D.: enRoute: dynamic path extraction from biological pathway maps for exploring heterogeneous experimental datasets. BMC Bioinformatics **14**(S19), S3 (2013). https://doi.org/10.1186/1471-2105-14-s19-s3
466. Parvin, B., Johnston, W., Roselli, D.: Pinta: a system for visualizing the anatomical structures of the brain from MR imaging. In: Proceeding of IEEE Conference on Computer Vision and Pattern Recognition, pp. 615–616 (1993). https://doi.org/10.1109/cvpr.1993.341059
467. Patel, M.V.: iS-CellR: a user-friendly tool for analyzing and visualizing single-cell RNA sequencing data. Bioinformatics **34**(24), 4305–4306 (2018). https://doi.org/10.1093/bioinformatics/bty517
468. Pedro, P.M., Amorim, J., Rojas, M.V., Sá, I.L., Galardo, A.K.R., Neto, N.F.S., de Carvalho, D.P., Ribeiro, K.A.N., Razzolini, M.T.P., Sallum, M.A.M.: Culicidae-centric metabarcoding through targeted use of D2 ribosomal DNA primers. PeerJ **8**, e9057 (2020). https://doi.org/10.7717/peerj.9057
469. Pei, Y., Xia, W., Wang, X., Li, J., Ye, H., Wang, L.: 3D structure surface modelling from volumetric CT images. In: Proceeding of IEEE International Symposium on Biomedical Imaging, pp. 476–479 (2019). https://doi.org/10.1109/ISBI.2019.8759432
470. Pelizzari, C., Grzeszczuk, R., Johnson, L., Ryan, M.: Distributed parallel volume rendering applied to virtual endoscopy. In: Proceeding of IEEE Engineering in Medicine and Biology, pp. 373–374 (1995). https://doi.org/10.1109/IEMBS.1995.575156
471. Pepe, A., Trotta, G.F., Gsaxner, C., Wallner, J., Egger, J., Schmalstieg, D., Bevilacqua, V.: Pattern recognition and mixed reality for computer-aided maxillofacial surgery and oncological assessment. In: Proceeding of Biomedical Engineering International Conference, pp. 1–5 (2018). https://doi.org/10.1109/bmeicon.2018.8609921
472. Peters, T., Davey, B., Munger, P., Comeau, R., Evans, A., Olivier, A.: Three-dimensional multimodal image-guidance for neurosurgery. IEEE Trans. Med. Imaging **15**(2), 121–128 (1996). https://doi.org/10.1109/42.491414
473. Pfister, H., Hardenbergh, J., Knittel, J., Lauer, H., Seiler, L.: The volumepro real-time ray-casting system. In: Proceeding of ACM SIGGRAPH, pp. 251–260 (1999). https://doi.org/10.1145/311535.311563

474. Pfister, H., Kaynig, V., Botha, C.P., Bruckner, S., Dercksen, V.J., Hege, H.C., Roerdink, J.B.: Visualization in connectomics. In: Scientific Visualization, pp. 221–245. Springer (2014). https://doi.org/10.1007/978-1-4471-6497-521
475. Phelan, I., Arden, M., Garcia, C., Roast, C.: Exploring virtual reality and prosthetic training. In: Proceeding of IEEE Virtual Reality, pp. 353–354 (2015). https://doi.org/10.1109/vr.2015.7223441
476. Pierpaoli, C., Basser, P.J.: Toward a quantitative assessment of diffusion anisotropy. Magn. Reson. Med. **36**(6), 893–906 (1996). https://doi.org/10.1002/mrm.1910360612
477. Plaisant, C., Mushlin, R., Snyder, A., Li, J., Heller, D., Shneiderman, B.: Lifelines: Using visualization to enhance navigation and analysis of patient records. In: The Craft of Information Visualization, pp. 308–312. Morgan Kaufmann (2003). https://doi.org/10.1016/b978-155860915-0/50038-x
478. Pohlandt, D., Preim, B., Saalfeld, P.: Supporting anatomy education with a 3D puzzle in a VR environment-results from a pilot study. In: Proceeding of Mensch und Computer, pp. 91–102 (2019). https://doi.org/10.1145/3340764.3340792
479. Pommert, A., Höhne, K.H.: Validation of medical volume visualization: a literature review. In: Proceeding of Computer-Assisted Radiology and Surgery, pp. 571–576 (2003). https://doi.org/10.1016/s0531-5131(03)00310-8
480. Pommert, A., Höhne, K.H., Pflesser, B., Richter, E., Riemer, M., Schiemann, T., Schubert, R., Schumacher, U., Tiede, U.: Creating a high-resolution spatial/symbolic model of the inner organs based on the Visible Human. Med. Image Anal. **5**(3), 221–228 (2001). https://doi.org/10.1016/S1361-8415(01)00044-5
481. Ponciano, D., Seefelder, M., Marroquim, R.: Graph-based interactive volume exploration. Comput. Graph. **60**, 55–65 (2016). https://doi.org/10.1016/j.cag.2016.06.007
482. Popescu, V.G., Burdea, G.C., Bouzit, M., Hentz, V.R.: A virtual-reality-based telerehabilitation system with force feedback. IEEE Trans. Inf Technol. Biomed. **4**(1), 45–51 (2000). https://doi.org/10.1109/4233.826858
483. Preim, B., Baer, A., Cunningham, D., Isenberg, T., Ropinski, T.: A survey of perceptually motivated 3D visualization of medical image data. Comput. Graph. Forum **35**(3), 501–525 (2016). https://doi.org/10.1111/CGF.12927
484. Preim, B., Bourquain, H., Selle, D., Oldhafer, K.: Resection proposals for oncologic liver surgery based on vascular territories. In: Proceeding of Computer Assisted Radiology and Surgery, pp. 353–358 (2002). https://doi.org/10.1007/978-3-642-56168-958
485. Preim, B., Lawonn, K.: A survey of visual analytics for public health. Comput. Graph. Forum **39**(1), 543–580 (2020). https://doi.org/10.1111/CGF.13891
486. Preim, B., Meuschke, M.: A survey of medical animations. Comput. Graph. **90**, 145–168 (2020). https://doi.org/10.1016/j.cag.2020.06.003
487. Preim, B., Oeltze, S., Mlejnek, M., Gröller, E., Hennemuth, A., Behrens, S.: Survey of the visual exploration and analysis of perfusion data. IEEE Trans. Vis. Comput. Graph. **15**(2), 205–220 (2008). https://doi.org/10.1109/TVCG.2008.95
488. Preim, B., Raidou, R.G., Smit, N.N., Lawonn, K.: Visualization, Visual Analytics and Virtual Reality in Medicine: State-of-the-art Techniques and Applications. Elsevier (2023). https://doi.org/10.1016/C2019-0-04604-3
489. Preim, B., Ropinski, T., Isenberg, P.: A critical analysis of the evaluation practice in medical visualization. In: Proceeding of Eurographics Workshop on Visual Computing for Biology and Medicine, pp. 45–56 (2018). https://doi.org/10.2312/VCBM.20181228
490. Preim, B., Saalfeld, P.: A survey of virtual human anatomy education systems. Comput. Graph. **71**, 132–153 (2018). https://doi.org/10.1016/j.cag.2018.01.005

491. Preim, B., Spindler, W., Oldhafer, K.J., Peitgen, H.O.: 3D-interaction techniques for planning of oncologic soft tissue operations. In: Proceeding of Graphics Interface, vol. 2001, pp. 183–190 (2001). https://doi.org/10.20380/GI2001.22
492. Preim, B., Tietjen, C., Spindler, W., Peitgen, H.: Integration of measurement tools in medical 3D visualizations. In: Proceeding of IEEE Visualization, pp. 21–28 (2002). https://doi.org/10.1109/VISUAL.2002.1183752
493. Principe, J.C., Yu, F., Reid, S.A.: Display of EEG chaotic dynamics. In: Proceeding of Visualization in Biomedical Computing, pp. 346–347 (1990). https://doi.org/10.1109/vbc.1990.109341
494. Procter, J.B., Thompson, J., Letunic, I., Creevey, C., Jossinet, F., Barton, G.J.: Visualization of multiple alignments, phylogenies and gene family evolution. Nat. Methods **7**(3), S16–S25 (2010). https://doi.org/10.1038/nmeth.1434
495. Pruim, R.J., Welch, R.P., Sanna, S., Teslovich, T.M., Chines, P.S., Gliedt, T.P., Boehnke, M., Abecasis, G.R., Willer, C.J.: LocusZoom: regional visualization of genome-wide association scan results. Bioinformatics **26**(18), 2336–2337 (2010). https://doi.org/10.1093/bioinformatics/btq419
496. Puig, A., Tost, D., Navazo, I.: An interactive cerebral blood vessel exploration system. In: Proceeding of IEEE Visualization, pp. 443–446 (1997). https://doi.org/10.1109/visual.1997.663917
497. Qiu, P., Simonds, E.F., Bendall, S.C., Gibbs, K.D., Bruggner, R.V., Linderman, M.D., Sachs, K., Nolan, G.P., Plevritis, S.K.: Extracting a cellular hierarchy from high-dimensional cytometry data with SPADE. Nat. Biotechnol. **29**(10), 886–891 (2011). https://doi.org/10.1038/nbt.1991
498. Quang, T., Zhou, M., Papay, F., Liu, Y.: Fluorescence to color feature-based image registration for medical augmented reality. In: Proceeding of IEEE International Symposium on Signal Processing and Information Technology, pp. 1–6 (2018). https://doi.org/10.1109/isspit.2018.8705148
499. Rahmadiva, M., Arifin, A., Fatoni, M.H., Baki, S.H., Watanabe, T.: A design of multipurpose virtual reality game for children with autism spectrum disorder. In: Proceeding of Biomedical Instrumentation and Technology Conference, vol. 1, pp. 1–6 (2019). https://doi.org/10.1109/ibitec46597.2019.9091713
500. Raidou, R.G., Casares-Magaz, O., Amirkhanov, A., Moiseenko, V., Muren, L.P., Einck, J.P., Vilanova, A., Gröller, M.E.: Bladder runner: visual analytics for the exploration of RT-induced bladder toxicity in a cohort study. Comput. Graph. Forum **37**(3), 205–216 (2018). https://doi.org/10.1111/CGF.13413
501. Raidou, R.G., Gröller, M.E., Wu, H.Y.: Slice and Dice: a physicalization workflow for anatomical edutainment. Comput. Graph. Forum **39**(7), 623–634 (2020). https://doi.org/10.1111/cgf.14173
502. Raidou, R.G., van der Heide, U.A., Dinh, C.V., Ghobadi, G., Kallehauge, J.F., Breeuwer, M., Vilanova, A.: Visual analytics for the exploration of tumor tissue characterization. Comput. Graph. Forum **34**(3), 11–20 (2015). https://doi.org/10.1111/CGF.12613
503. Raidou, R.G., Kuijf, H.J., Sepasian, N., Pezzotti, N., Bouvy, W.H., Breeuwer, M., Vilanova, A.: Employing visual analytics to aid the design of white matter hyperintensity classifiers. In: International Conference on Medical Image Computing and Computer-Assisted Intervention, pp. 97–105 (2016). https://doi.org/10.1007/978-3-319-46723-812
504. Reina, G., Childs, H., Matković, K., Bühler, K., Waldner, M., Pugmire, D., Kozlíková, B., Ropinski, T., Ljung, P., Itoh, T., et al.: The moving target of visualization software for an increasingly complex world. Comput. Graph. **87**, 12–29 (2020). https://doi.org/10.1016/j.cag.2020.01.005

505. Reiter, O., Breeuwer, M., Gröller, E., Raidou, R.G.: Comparative visual analysis of pelvic organ segmentation. In: Proceeding of EuroVis—Short Papers, pp. 37–41 (2018). https://doi.org/10.2312/eurovisshort.20181075
506. Rengier, F., Mehndiratta, A., Von Tengg-Kobligk, H., Zechmann, C., Unterhinninghofen, R., Kauczor, H.U., Giesel, F.: 3D printing based on imaging data: review of medical applications. Int. J. Comput. Assist. Radiol. Surg. **5**, 335–341 (2010). https://doi.org/10.1007/s11548-010-0476-x
507. Reniers, D., Jalba, A., Telea, A.: Robust classification and analysis of anatomical surfaces using 3D skeletons. In: Proceeding of Eurographics Workshop on Visual Computing in Biology and Medicine, pp. 61–68 (2008). https://doi.org/10.2312/VCBM/VCBM08/061-068 In: Proceeding
508. Rezk-Salama, C., Kolb, A.: Opacity peeling for direct volume rendering. Comput. Graph. Forum **25**(3), 597–606 (2006). https://doi.org/10.1111/j.1467-8659.2006.00979.x
509. Ribeiro, V.S., Santana, C.A., Fassio, A.V., Cerqueira, F.R., da Silveira, C.H., Romanelli, J.P.R., Patarroyo-Vargas, A., Oliveira, M.G.A., Gonçalves-Almeida, V., Izidoro, S.C., de Melo-Minardi, R.C., de A. Silveira, S.: visGReMLIN: graph mining-based detection and visualization of conserved motifs at 3D protein-ligand interface at the atomic level. BMC Bioinformatics **21**(S2), 80 (2020). https://doi.org/10.1186/s12859-020-3347-7
510. Richards, F.M.: Areas, volumes, packing, and protein structure. Annu. Rev. Biophys. Bioeng. **6**(1), 151–176 (1977). https://doi.org/10.1146/annurev.bb.06.060177.001055
511. Richardson, J.S.: The anatomy and taxonomy of protein structure. Adv. Protein Chem. **34**, 167–339 (1981). https://doi.org/10.1016/s0065-3233(08)60520-3
512. Riches, S., Azevedo, L., Bird, L., Pisani, S., Valmaggia, L.: Virtual reality relaxation for the general population: a systematic review. Soc. Psychiatry Psychiatr. Epidemiol. **56**(10), 1707–1727 (2021). https://doi.org/10.1007/s00127-021-02110-z
513. Rieder, C., Ritter, F., Raspe, M., Peitgen, H.O.: Interactive visualization of multimodal volume data for neurosurgical tumor treatment. Comput. Graph. Forum **27**(3), 1055–1062 (2008). https://doi.org/10.1111/J.1467-8659.2008.01242.X
514. Rieder, C., Schwier, M., Hahn, H.K., Peitgen, H.O.: High-quality multimodal volume visualization of intracerebral pathological tissue. In: Proceeding of Eurographics Workshop on Visual Computing in Biology and Medicine, pp. 167–176 (2008). https://doi.org/10.2312/VCBM/VCBM08/167-176
515. Rieder, C., Weihusen, A., Schumann, C., Zidowitz, S., Peitgen, H.O.: Visual support for interactive post-interventional assessment of radiofrequency ablation therapy. Comput. Graph. Forum **29**(3), 1093–1102 (2010). https://doi.org/10.1111/J.1467-8659.2009.01665.X
516. Riener, R., Frey, M., Proll, T., Regenfelder, F., Burgkart, R.: Phantom-based multimodal interactions for medical education and training: the Munich knee joint simulator. IEEE Trans. Inf Technol. Biomed. **8**(2), 208–216 (2004). https://doi.org/10.1109/titb.2004.828885
517. Ristovski, G., Garbers, N., Hahn, H.K., Preusser, T., Linsen, L.: Uncertainty-aware visual analysis of radiofrequency ablation simulations. Comput. Graph. **79**, 24–35 (2019). https://doi.org/10.1016/j.cag.2018.12.005
518. Ristovski, G., Preusser, T., Hahn, H.K., Linsen, L.: Uncertainty in medical visualization: towards a taxonomy. Comput. Graph. **39**, 60–73 (2014). https://doi.org/10.1016/j.cag.2013.10.015
519. Ritter, F., Hansen, C., Dicken, V., Konrad, O., Preim, B., Peitgen, H.O.: Real-time illustration of vascular structures. IEEE Trans. Vis. Comput. Graph. **12**(5), 877–884 (2006). https://doi.org/10.1109/tvcg.2006.172
520. Rizzo, A.S., Difede, J., Rothbaum, B., Reger, G., Spitalnick, J., Cukor, J., Mclay, R.: Development and early evaluation of the virtual Iraq/Afghanistan exposure therapy system for combat-related PTSD. Ann. N. Y. Acad. Sci. **1208**(1), 114–125 (2010). https://doi.org/10.1111/j.1749-6632.2010.05755.x

521. Robinson, A., MacEachren, A., Roth, R.: Designing a web-based learning portal for geographic visualization and analysis in public health. Health Inf. J. **17**(3), 191–208 (2011). https://doi.org/10.1177/1460458211409718
522. Roederer, M., Moody, M.A.: Polychromatic plots: graphical display of multidimensional data. Cytometry A **73A**(9), 868–874 (2008). https://doi.org/10.1002/cyto.a.20610
523. Rojdestenski, I., Modjeska, D., Pettersson, F., Rojdestvenskaia, M., Gustafsson, P.: Sequence-World: a genetics database in virtual reality. In: Proceeding of IEEE Conference on Information Visualization, pp. 513–517 (2000). https://doi.org/10.1109/IV.2000.859805
524. Roos, J.E., Fleischmann, D., Köchl, A., Rakshe, T., Straka, M., Napoli, A., Kanitsar, A., Sramek, M., Gröller, E.: Multipath curved planar reformation of the peripheral arterial tree in CT angiography. Radiology **244**(1), 281–290 (2007). https://doi.org/10.1148/radiol.2441060976
525. Ropinski, T., Meyer-Spradow, J., Diepenbrock, S., Mensmann, J., Hinrichs, K.: Interactive volume rendering with dynamic ambient occlusion and color bleeding. Comput. Graph. Forum **27**(2), 567–576 (2008). https://doi.org/10.1111/j.1467-8659.2008.01154.x
526. Ropinski, T., Oeltze, S., Preim, B.: Survey of glyph-based visualization techniques for spatial multivariate medical data. Comput. Graph. **35**(2), 392–401 (2011). https://doi.org/10.1016/j.cag.2011.01.011
527. Ropinski, T., Steinicke, F., Hinrichs, K.: Visually supporting depth perception in angiography imaging. In: Proceeding of International Symposium on Smart Graphics, pp. 93–104 (2006). https://doi.org/10.1007/117950189
528. Rössling, I., Dornheim, J., Dornheim, L., Boehm, A., Preim, B.: The tumor therapy manager—design, refinement and clinical use of a software product for ENT surgery planning and documentation. In: Proceeding of Information Processing in Computer-Assisted Interventions, pp. 1–12 (2011)https://doi.org/10.1007/978-3-642-21504-91
529. Rothbaum, B., Hodges, L., Alarcon, R., Ready, D., Shahar, F., Graap, K., Pair, J., Hebert, P., et al.: Virtual reality exposure therapy for PTSD Vietnam veterans: a case study. J. Trauma. Stress **12**(2), 263–271 (1999). https://doi.org/10.1023/A:1024772308758
530. Rothbaum, B., Hodges, L., Kooper, R., Opdyke, D., Williford, J., North, M.: Effectiveness of computer-generated (virtual reality) graded exposure in the treatment of acrophobia. Am. J. Psychiatry **152**(4), 626–628 (1995). https://doi.org/10.1176/ajp.152.4.626
531. Rozario, S.V., Housman, S., Kovic, M., Kenyon, R.V., Patton, J.L.: Therapist-mediated post-stroke rehabilitation using haptic/graphic error augmentation. In: Proceeding of IEEE Engineering in Medicine and Biology, pp. 1151–1156 (2009). https://doi.org/10.1109/iembs.2009.5333875
532. Rubel, O., Weber, G., Huang, M.Y., Bethel, E., Biggin, M., Fowlkes, C., Hendriks, C.L., Keranen, S., Eisen, M., Knowles, D., Malik, J., Hagen, H., Hamann, B.: Integrating data clustering and visualization for the analysis of 3D gene expression data. IEEE/ACM Trans. Comput. Biol. Bioinf. **7**(1), 64–79 (2010). https://doi.org/10.1109/tcbb.2008.49
533. Russ, C., Kubisch, C., Qiu, F., Hong, W., Ljung, P.: Real-time surface analysis and tagged material cleansing for virtual colonoscopy. In: Proceeding of Volume Graphics at Eurographics, pp. 29–36 (2010). https://doi.org/10.2312/VG/VG10/029-036
534. Saalfeld, P., Stojnic, A., Preim, B., Oeltze-Jafra, S.: Semi-immersive 3D sketching of vascular structures for medical education. In: Proceeding of Eurographics Workshop on Visual Computing for Biology and Medicine, pp. 123–132 (2016). https://doi.org/10.2312/vcbm.20161280
535. Sabando, M.V., Ulbrich, P., Selzer, M., Byška, J., Mičan, J., Ponzoni, I., Soto, A.J., Ganuza, M.L., Kozlíková, B.: ChemVA: interactive visual analysis of chemical compound similarity in virtual screening. IEEE Trans. Vis. Comput. Graph. **27**(2), 891–901 (2021). https://doi.org/10.1109/tvcg.2020.3030438
536. Sakai, R., Aerts, J.: Sequence diversity diagram for comparative analysis of multiple sequence alignments. BMC Proc. **8**(2), S9 (2014). https://doi.org/10.1186/1753-6561-8-S2-S9

537. Sakas, G.: Trends in medical imaging: from 2D to 3D. Comput. Graph. **26**(4), 577–587 (2002). https://doi.org/10.1016/S0097-8493(02)00103-6
538. Sakas, G., Pommert, A.: Advanced applications of volume visualization methods in medicine. In: Proceeding of Eurographics—STARs, pp. 1–43 (1997). https://doi.org/10.2312/egst.19971004
539. Samusik, N., Good, Z., Spitzer, M.H., Davis, K.L., Nolan, G.P.: Automated mapping of phenotype space with single-cell data. Nat. Methods **13**(6), 493–496 (2016). https://doi.org/10.1038/nmeth.3863
540. Santamaría, R., Therón, R., Quintales, L.: A visual analytics approach for understanding biclustering results from microarray data. BMC Bioinformatics **9**(1), 247 (2008). https://doi.org/10.1186/1471-2105-9-247
541. Sato, Y., Nakamoto, M., Tamaki, Y., Sasama, T., Sakita, I., Nakajima, Y., Monden, M., Tamura, S.: Image guidance of breast cancer surgery using 3-D ultrasound images and augmented reality visualization. IEEE Trans. Med. Imaging **17**(5), 681–693 (1998). https://doi.org/10.1109/42.736019
542. Sayle, R.A., Milner-White, E.J.: RASMOL: biomolecular graphics for all. Trends Biochem. Sci. **20**(9), 374–376 (1995). https://doi.org/10.1016/s0968-0004(00)89080-5
543. Schapiro, D., Jackson, H.W., Raghuraman, S., Fischer, J.R., Zanotelli, V.R.T., Schulz, D., Giesen, C., Catena, R., Varga, Z., Bodenmiller, B.: histoCAT: analysis of cell phenotypes and interactions in multiplex image cytometry data. Nat. Methods **14**(9), 873–876 (2017). https://doi.org/10.1038/nmeth.4391
544. Schatz, K., Frieß, F., Schäfer, M., Buchholz, P.C., Pleiss, J., Ertl, T., Krone, M.: Analyzing the similarity of protein domains by clustering molecular surface maps. Comput. Graph. **99**, 114–127 (2021). https://doi.org/10.1016/j.cag.2021.06.007
545. Schatz, K., Krone, M., Bauer, T.L., Ferrario, V., Pleiss, J., Ertl, T.: Molecular Sombreros: Abstract visualization of binding sites within proteins. In: Proceeding of Eurographics Workshop on Visual Computing for Biology and Medicine, pp. 225–237 (2019). https://doi.org/10.2312/VCBM.20191248
546. Schein, S., Elber, G.: Adaptive extraction and visualization of silhouette curves from volumetric datasets. Vis. Comput. **20**(4), 243–252 (2004). https://doi.org/10.1007/s00371-003-0230-2
547. Schindler, M., Korpitsch, T., Raidou, R.G., Wu, H.: Nested papercrafts for anatomical and biological edutainment. Comput. Graph. Forum **41**(3), 541–553 (2022). https://doi.org/10.1111/CGF.14561
548. Schindler, M., Wu, H.Y., Raidou, R.G.: The anatomical edutainer. In: Proceeding of IEEE Vis—Short Papers, pp. 1–5 (2020). https://doi.org/10.1109/VIS47514.2020.00007
549. Schlachter, M., Fechter, T., Adebahr, S., Schimek-Jasch, T., Nestle, U., Bühler, K.: Visualization of 4D multimodal imaging data and its applications in radiotherapy planning. J. Appl. Clin. Med. Phys. **18**(6), 183–193 (2017). https://doi.org/10.1002/acm2.12209
550. Schlachter, M., Fechter, T., Jurisic, M., Schimek-Jasch, T., Oehlke, O., Adebahr, S., Birkfellner, W., Nestle, U., Bühler, K.: Visualization of deformable image registration quality using local image dissimilarity. IEEE Trans. Med. Imaging **35**(10), 2319–2328 (2016). https://doi.org/10.1109/tmi.2016.2560942
551. Schlachter, M., Raidou, R.G., Muren, L.P., Preim, B., Putora, P.M., Bühler, K.: State-of-the-art report: visual computing in radiation therapy planning. Comput. Graph. Forum **38**(3), 753–779 (2019). https://doi.org/10.1111/cgf.13726
552. Schneider, T.D., Stephens, R.: Sequence logos: a new way to display consensus sequences. Nucleic Acids Res. **18**(20), 6097–6100 (1990). https://doi.org/10.1093/nar/18.20.6097
553. Schott, M., Pascal Grosset, A., Martin, T., Pegoraro, V., Smith, S.T., Hansen, C.D.: Depth of field effects for interactive direct volume rendering. Comput. Graph. Forum **30**(3), 941–950 (2011). https://doi.org/10.1111/j.1467-8659.2011.01943.x

554. Schreiber, F., Dwyer, T., Marriott, K., Wybrow, M.: A generic algorithm for layout of biological networks. BMC Bioinformatics **10**(1), 375 (2009). https://doi.org/10.1186/1471-2105-10-375
555. Schreiber, F., Schwobbermeyer, H.: MAVisto: a tool for the exploration of network motifs. Bioinformatics **21**(17), 3572–3574 (2005). https://doi.org/10.1093/bioinformatics/bti556
556. Schultz, T., Schlaffke, L., Schölkopf, B., Schmidt-Wilcke, T.: HiFiVE: a Hilbert space embedding of fiber variability estimates for uncertainty modeling and visualization. Comput. Graph. Forum **32**(3), 121–130 (2013). https://doi.org/10.1111/CGF.12099
557. Schultz, T., Vilanova, A.: Diffusion MRI visualization. NMR Biomed. **32**(4), e3902 (2019). https://doi.org/10.1002/nbm.3902
558. Schultz, T., Vilanova, A., Brecheisen, R., Kindlmann, G.: Fuzzy fibers: uncertainty in dMRI tractography. In: Scientific Visualization, pp. 79–92. Springer (2014). https://doi.org/10.1007/978-1-4471-6497-58
559. Schumann, C., Oeltze, S., Bade, R., Preim, B., Peitgen, H.O.: Model-free surface visualization of vascular trees. In: Proceeding of EuroVis, pp. 283–290 (2007)https://doi.org/10.2312/VISSYM/EUROVIS07/283-290
560. Schwartz, E.L., Merker, B.: Computer-aided neuroanatomy: differential geometry of cortical surfaces and an optimal flattening algorithm. IEEE Comput. Graph. Appl. **6**(3), 36–44 (1986). https://doi.org/10.1109/mcg.1986.276630
561. Sedig, K., Parsons, P., Dittmer, M., Ola, O.: Beyond information access: Support for complex cognitive activities in public health informatics tools. Online J. Public Health Inform. **4**(3) (2012). https://doi.org/10.5210/ojphi.v4i3.4270
562. Sehnal, D., Bittrich, S., Deshpande, M., Svobodová, R., Berka, K., Bazgier, V., Velankar, S., Burley, S.K., Koča, J., Rose, A.S.: Mol* Viewer: modern web app for 3D visualization and analysis of large biomolecular structures. Nucleic Acids Res. **49**(W1), W431–W437 (2021). https://doi.org/10.1093/NAR/GKAB314
563. Selle, D., Preim, B., Schenk, A., Peitgen, H.O.: Analysis of vasculature for liver surgical planning. IEEE Trans. Med. Imaging **21**(11), 1344–1357 (2002). https://doi.org/10.1109/tmi.2002.801166
564. Selver, M.A.: Exploring brushlet based 3D textures in transfer function specification for direct volume rendering of abdominal organs. IEEE Trans. Vis. Comput. Graph. **21**(2), 174–187 (2015). https://doi.org/10.1109/TVCG.2014.2359462
565. Setty, M., Kiseliovas, V., Levine, J., Gayoso, A., Mazutis, L., Pe'er, D.: Characterization of cell fate probabilities in single-cell data with Palantir. Nat. Biotechnol. **37**(4), 451–460 (2019). https://doi.org/10.1038/s41587-019-0068-4
566. Shahidi, R., Lorensen, B., Kikinis, R., Flynn, J., Kaufman, A., Napel, S.: Surface rendering versus volume rendering in medical imaging: techniques and applications. In: Proceeding of IEEE Visualization, pp. 439–440 (1996). https://doi.org/10.1109/VISUAL.1996.568151
567. Shamir, R.R., Horn, M., Blum, T., Mehrkens, J., Shoshan, Y., Joskowicz, L., Navab, N.: Trajectory planning with augmented reality for improved risk assessment in image-guided keyhole neurosurgery. In: Proceeding of IEEE International Symposium on Biomedical Imaging: From Nano to Macro, pp. 1873–1876 (2011). https://doi.org/10.1109/isbi.2011.5872773
568. Shannon, P., Markiel, A., Ozier, O., Baliga, N.S., Wang, J.T., Ramage, D., Amin, N., Schwikowski, B., Ideker, T.: Cytoscape: a software environment for integrated models of biomolecular interaction networks. Genome Res. **13**(11), 2498–2504 (2003). https://doi.org/10.1101/gr.1239303
569. Sharko, J., Grinstein, G.G., Marx, K.A., Zhou, J., Cheng, C.H., Odelberg, S., Simon, H.G.: Heat map visualizations allow comparison of multiple clustering results and evaluation of dataset quality: Application to microarray data. In: Proceeding of IEEE Conference on Information Visualization (2007). https://doi.org/10.1109/iv.2007.61

570. Shaw, C.D., Dasch, G.A., Eremeeva, M.E.: IMAS: the interactive multigenomic analysis system. In: Proceeding of IEEE Symposium on Visual Analytics Science and Technology, pp. 59–66 (2007). https://doi.org/10.1109/VAST.2007.4388997
571. Shekhar, K., Brodin, P., Davis, M.M., Chakraborty, A.K.: Automatic classification of cellular expression by nonlinear stochastic embedding (ACCENSE). Proc. Natl. Acad. Sci. **111**(1), 202–207 (2013). https://doi.org/10.1073/pnas.1321405111
572. Shen, R., Boulanger, P., Noga, M.: MedVis: A real-time immersive visualization environment for the exploration of medical volumetric data. In: Proceeding of MediVis BioMedical Visualization, pp. 63–68 (2008). https://doi.org/10.1109/MediVis.2008.10
573. Shenton, M., Kikinis, R., McCarley, W., Saiviroonporn, P., Hokama, H., Robatino, A., Metcalf, D., Wible, C., Portas, C., Iosifescu, D., et al.: Harvard brain atlas: a teaching and visualization tool. In: Proceeding of Biomedical Visualization, pp. 10–17 (1995). https://doi.org/10.1109/biovis.1995.528700
574. Shieu, D., Athey, B., Anderson, D.: An efficient surface rendering technique utilizing Fourier descriptors to visualize three dimensional biomedical image data sets. In: Proceeding of Midwest Symposium on Circuits and Systems, vol. 2, pp. 1247–1250 (1993). https://doi.org/10.1109/MWSCAS.1993.343323
575. Shih, A.C.C., Lee, D., Lin, L., Peng, C.L., Chen, S.H., Wong, C.Y., Chou, M.Y., Shiao, T.C.: SinicView: an interactive visualization tool for comparison of multiple sequence alignment results. In: Proceeding of IEEE Computational Systems Bioinformatics Conference—Workshops, pp. 269–270 (2005). https://doi.org/10.1109/CSBW.2005.127
576. Shin-Ting, W., Yasuda, C.L., Cendes, F.: Interactive curvilinear reformatting in native space. IEEE Trans. Vis. Comput. Graph. **18**(2), 299–308 (2011). https://doi.org/10.1109/TVCG.2011.40
577. Shneiderman, B., Plaisant, C.: Strategies for evaluating information visualization tools: multidimensional in-depth long-term case studies. In: Proceeding of the AVI Workshop on BEyond Time and Errors: Novel Evaluation Methods for Information Visualization, pp. 1–7 (2006). https://doi.org/10.1145/1168149.1168158
578. Sielhorst, T., Feuerstein, M., Navab, N.: Advanced medical displays: a literature review of augmented reality. J. Display Technol. **4**(4), 451–467 (2008). https://doi.org/10.1109/JDT.2008.2001575
579. Simões, T.M., Gomes, A.J.: CavVis-a field-of-view geometric algorithm for protein cavity detection. J. Chem. Inf. Model. **59**(2), 786–796 (2019). https://doi.org/10.1021/ACS.JCIM.8B00572
580. Simon, S., Oelke, D., Landstorfer, R., Neuhaus, K., Keim, D.A.: Visual analysis of next-generation sequencing data to detect overlapping genes in bacterial genomes. In: Proceeding of IEEE Symposium on Biological Data Visualization (2011). https://doi.org/10.1109/biovis.2011.6094047
581. Sinha, A.U., Meller, J.: Cinteny: flexible analysis and visualization of synteny and genome rearrangements in multiple organisms. BMC Bioinformatics **8**(1), 82 (2007). https://doi.org/10.1186/1471-2105-8-82
582. Skånberg, R., Vázquez, P.P., Guallar, V., Ropinski, T.: Real-time molecular visualization supporting diffuse interreflections and ambient occlusion. IEEE Trans. Vis. Comput. Graph. **22**(1), 718–727 (2015). https://doi.org/10.1109/TVCG.2015.2467293
583. Skånberg, R., Linares, M., König, C., Norman, P., Jönsson, D., Hotz, I., Ynnerman, A.: VIA-MD: Visual interactive analysis of molecular dynamics. In: Proceeding of Workshop on Molecular Graphics and Visual Analysis of Molecular Data, pp. 19–27 (2018). https://doi.org/10.2312/MOLVA.20181102

584. Smelyanskiy, M., Holmes, D., Chhugani, J., Larson, A., Carmean, D.M., Hanson, D., Dubey, P., Augustine, K., Kim, D., Kyker, A., Lee, V.W., Nguyen, A.D., Seiler, L., Robb, R.: Mapping high-fidelity volume rendering for medical imaging to CPU, GPU and many-core architectures. IEEE Trans. Vis. Comput. Graph. **15**(6), 1563–1570 (2009). https://doi.org/10.1109/TVCG.2009.164
585. Smit, N.N., Haneveld, B.K., Staring, M., Eisemann, E., Botha, C.P., Vilanova, A.: RegistrationShop: an interactive 3D medical volume registration system. In: Proceeding of Eurographics Workshop on Visual Computing for Biology and Medicine, pp. 145–153 (2014). https://doi.org/10.2312/vcbm.20141193
586. Smit, N.N., Hofstede, C.W., Kraima, A., Jansma, D., deRuiter, M., Eisemann, E., Vilanova, A.: The online anatomical human: web-based anatomy education. In: Proceeding of EuroGraphics: Education Papers, pp. 37–40 (2016). https://doi.org/10.2312/eged.20161025
587. Smit, N.N., Lawonn, K., Kraima, A., DeRuiter, M., Sokooti, H., Bruckner, S., Eisemann, E., Vilanova, A.: Pelvis: atlas-based surgical planning for oncological pelvic surgery. IEEE Trans. Vis. Comput. Graph. **23**(1), 741–750 (2016). https://doi.org/10.1109/tvcg.2016.2598826
588. Smith, G.M., Gund, P.: Computer-generated space-filling molecular models. J. Chem. Inf. Comput. Sci. **18**(4), 207–210 (1978). https://doi.org/10.1021/CI60016A006
589. Somarakis, A., Ijsselsteijn, M.E., Kenkhuis, B., Unen, V.v., Luk, S.J., Koning, F., Weerd, L.v.d., Miranda, N.F.C.C.d., Lelieveldt, B.P.F., Höllt, T.: Visual analysis of tissue images at cellular level. In: Proceeding of EuroVis—Dirk Bartz Prize, pp. 1–5 (2021). https://doi.org/10.2312/evm.20211074
590. Somarakis, A., Ijsselsteijn, M.E., Luk, S.J., Kenkhuis, B., de Miranda, N.F., Lelieveldt, B.P., Höllt, T.: Visual cohort comparison for spatial single-cell omics-data. IEEE Trans. Vis. Comput. Graph. **27**(2), 733–743 (2021). https://doi.org/10.1109/tvcg.2020.3030336
591. Somarakis, A., Unen, V.V., Koning, F., Lelieveldt, B., Höllt, T.: ImaCytE: visual exploration of cellular micro-environments for imaging mass cytometry data. IEEE Trans. Vis. Comput. Graph. **27**(1), 98–110 (2021). https://doi.org/10.1109/tvcg.2019.2931299
592. Sorger, J., Bühler, K., Schulze, F., Liu, T., Dickson, B.: neuroMAP-Interactive graph-visualization of the fruit fly's neural circuit. In: Proceeding of IEEE Symposium on Biological Data Visualization, pp. 73–80 (2013). https://doi.org/10.1109/biovis.2013.6664349
593. Sousa, M.C., Ebert, D.S., Stredney, D., Svakhine, N.A.: Illustrative visualization for medical training. In: Proceeding of Eurographics Conference on Computational Aesthetics in Graphics, Visualization and Imaging, pp. 201–208 (2005). https://doi.org/10.2312/COMPAESTH/COMPAESTH05/201-208
594. Specht, M., Lebrun, R., Zollikofer, C.P.: Visualizing shape transformation between chimpanzee and human braincases. Vis. Comput. **23**(9), 743–751 (2007). https://doi.org/10.1007/S00371-007-0156-1
595. Spell, R., Brady, R., Dierich, F.: BARD: a visualization tool for biological sequence analysis. In: Proceeding of IEEE Symposium on Information Visualization, pp. 219–225 (2003). https://doi.org/10.1109/INFVIS.2003.1249029
596. Stefan, P., Habert, S., Winkler, A., Lazarovici, M., Fürmetz, J., Eck, U., Navab, N.: A radiation-free mixed-reality training environment and assessment concept for c-arm-based surgery. Int. J. Comput. Assist. Radiol. Surg. **13**(9), 1335–1344 (2018). https://doi.org/10.1007/s11548-018-1807-6
597. Stellman, S.D.: Application of three-dimensional interactive graphics in X-ray crystallographic analysis. Comput. Graph. **1**(2), 279–288 (1975). https://doi.org/10.1016/0097-8493(75)90019-9
598. Stoltzfus, C.R., Filipek, J., Gern, B.H., Olin, B.E., Leal, J.M., Wu, Y., Lyons-Cohen, M.R., Huang, J.Y., Paz-Stoltzfus, C.L., Plumlee, C.R., Pöschinger, T., Urdahl, K.B., Perro, M., Gerner,

M.Y.: CytoMAP: a spatial analysis toolbox reveals features of myeloid cell organization in lymphoid tissues. Cell Rep. **31**(3), 107523 (2020). https://doi.org/10.1016/j.celrep.2020.107523

599. Stoppel, S., Bruckner, S.: Vol2velle: printable interactive volume visualization. IEEE Trans. Vis. Comput. Graph. **23**(01), 861–870 (2017). https://doi.org/10.1109/TVCG.2016.2599211
600. Streit, M., Ecker, R.C., Österreicher, K., Steiner, G.E., Bischof, H., Bangert, C., Kopp, T., Rogojanu, R.: 3D parallel coordinate systems-A new data visualization method in the context of microscopy-based multicolor tissue cytometry. Cytometry A **69A**(7), 601–611 (2006). https://doi.org/10.1002/cyto.a.20288
601. Streit, M., Kalkusch, M., Kashofer, K., Schmalstieg, D.: Navigation and exploration of interconnected pathways. Comput. Graph. Forum **27**(3), 951–958 (2008). https://doi.org/10.1111/j.1467-8659.2008.01229.x
602. Sugathan, S., Bartsch, H., Riemer, F., Grüner, R., Lawonn, K., Smit, N.N.: Interactive multimodal imaging visualization for multiple sclerosis lesion analysis. In: Proceeding of Eurographics Workshop on Visual Computing for Biology and Medicine, pp. 65–77 (2021). https://doi.org/10.2312/vcbm.20211346
603. Sultanum, N., Singh, D., Brudno, M., Chevalier, F.: Doccurate: a curation-based approach for clinical text visualization. IEEE Trans. Vis. Comput. Graph. **25**(1), 142–151 (2018). https://doi.org/10.1109/TVCG.2018.2864905
604. Svakhine, N.A., Ebert, D.S., Andrews, W.M.: Illustration-inspired depth enhanced volumetric medical visualization. IEEE Trans. Vis. Comput. Graph. **15**(1), 77–86 (2009). https://doi.org/10.1109/TVCG.2008.56
605. Svakhine, N.A., Ebert, D.S., Stredney, D.: Illustration motifs for effective medical volume illustration. IEEE Comput. Graph. Appl. **25**(3), 31–39 (2005). https://doi.org/10.1109/mcg.2005.60
606. Svetachov, P., Everts, M.H., Isenberg, T.: DTI in context: illustrating brain fiber tracts in situ. Comput. Graph. Forum **29**(3), 1023–1032 (2010). https://doi.org/10.1111/J.1467-8659.2009.01692.X
607. Swamy, N.K.L., Chavan, P.S., Murthy, S.: StereoChem: augmented reality 3D molecular model visualization app for teaching and learning stereochemistry. In: Proceeding of IEEE International Conference on Advanced Learning Technologies, pp. 252–256 (2018). https://doi.org/10.1109/icalt.2018.00065
608. Talbot, H., Haouchine, N., Peterlik, I., Dequidt, J., Duriez, C., Delingette, H., Cotin, S.: Surgery training, planning and guidance using the sofa framework. In: Proceeding of Eurographics—Dirk Bartz Prize, pp. 1–4 (2015). https://doi.org/10.2312/EGM.20151028
609. Tanabashi, S.: STE (A) M education of cell biology using advanced 3D technology for K-12 learning. In: Proceeding of IEEE Teaching, Assessment, and Learning for Engineering, pp. 922–924 (2020). https://doi.org/10.1109/tale48869.2020.9368441
610. Tappenbeck, A., Preim, B., Dicken, V.: Distance-based transfer function design: Specification methods and applications. In: Proceeding of SimVis, pp. 259–274 (2006)
611. Tarini, M., Cignoni, P., Montani, C.: Ambient occlusion and edge cueing for enhancing real time molecular visualization. IEEE Trans. Vis. Comput. Graph. **12**(5), 1237–1244 (2006). https://doi.org/10.1109/TVCG.2006.115
612. Taubin, G.: Curve and surface smoothing without shrinkage. In: Proceeding of IEEE International Conference on Computer Vision, pp. 852–857 (1995). https://doi.org/10.1109/iccv.1995.466848
613. Taylor, W.R.: The classification of amino acid conservation. J. Theor. Biol. **119**(2), 205–218 (1986). https://doi.org/10.1016/S0022-5193(86)80075-3
614. Ten Caat, M., Maurits, N.M., Roerdink, J.B.: Design and evaluation of tiled parallel coordinate visualization of multichannel EEG data. IEEE Trans. Vis. Comput. Graph. **13**(1), 70–79 (2006). https://doi.org/10.1109/tvcg.2007.9

615. Ten Caat, M., Maurits, N.M., Roerdink, J.B.: Data-driven visualization and group analysis of multichannel EEG coherence with functional units. IEEE Trans. Vis. Comput. Graph. **14**(4), 756–771 (2008). https://doi.org/10.1109/tvcg.2008.21
616. Termeer, M., Bescós, J.O., Breeuwer, M., Vilanova, A., Gerritsen, F., Gröller, E.: CoViCAD: comprehensive visualization of coronary artery disease. IEEE Trans. Vis. Comput. Graph. **13**(6), 1632–1639 (2007). https://doi.org/10.1109/tvcg.2007.70550
617. Termeer, M., Bescós, J.O., Breeuwer, M., Vilanova, A., Gerritsen, F.A., Gröller, M.E., Nagel, E.: Visualization of myocardial perfusion derived from coronary anatomy. IEEE Trans. Vis. Comput. Graph. **14**(6), 1595–1602 (2008). https://doi.org/10.1109/TVCG.2008.180
618. Thiagarajan, P., Gao, G.: Visualizing biosequence data using texture mapping. In: Proceeding of IEEE Symposium on Information Visualization, pp. 103–109 (2002). https://doi.org/10.1109/INFVIS.2002.1173154
619. Thomas, R.G., William John, N., Delieu, J.M.: Augmented reality for anatomical education. J. Vis. Commun. Med. **33**(1), 6–15 (2010). https://doi.org/10.3109/17453050903557359
620. Tiede, U., Höhne, K.H., Bomans, M., Pommert, A., Riemer, M., Wiebecke, G.: Investigation of medical 3D-rendering algorithms. IEEE Comput. Graph. Appl. **10**(2), 41–53 (1990). https://doi.org/10.1109/38.50672
621. Tiede, U., Schiemann, T., Höhne, K.H.: High quality rendering of attributed volume data. In: Proceeding of IEEE Visualization, pp. 255–262 (1998). https://doi.org/10.1109/visual.1998.745311
622. Tietjen, C., Isenberg, T., Preim, B.: Combining silhouettes, surface, and volume rendering for surgery education and planning. In: Proceeding of EuroVis, pp. 303–310 (2005). https://doi.org/10.2312/VisSym/EuroVis05/303-310
623. Tjoa, E., Guan, C.: A survey on explainable artificial intelligence (XAI): Toward medical XAI. IEEE Trans. Neural Netw. Learn. Syst. **32**(11), 4793–4813 (2021). https://doi.org/10.1109/TNNLS.2020.3027314
624. Torsney-Weir, T., Saad, A., Möller, T., Hege, H.C., Weber, B., Verbavatz, J.M., Bergner, S.: Tuner: principled parameter finding for image segmentation algorithms using visual response surface exploration. IEEE Trans. Vis. Comput. Graph. **17**(12), 1892–1901 (2011). https://doi.org/10.1109/tvcg.2011.248
625. Tory, M., Potts, S., Möller, T.: A parallel coordinates style interface for exploratory volume visualization. IEEE Trans. Vis. Comput. Graph. **11**(1), 71–80 (2005). https://doi.org/10.1109/TVCG.2005.2
626. Troidl, J., Cali, C., Gröller, E., Pfister, H., Hadwiger, M., Beyer, J.: Barrio: customizable spatial neighborhood analysis and comparison for nanoscale brain structures. Comput. Graph. Forum **41**, 183–194 (2022). https://doi.org/10.1111/CGF.14532
627. Tvarusko, W., Bentele, M., Misteli, T., Rudolf, R., Kaether, C., Spector, D.L., Gerdes, H., Eils, R.: Time-resolved analysis and visualization of dynamic processes in living cells. Proc. Natl. Acad. Sci. **96**(14), 7950–7955 (1999). https://doi.org/10.1073/pnas.96.14.7950
628. Ullrich, S., Kuhlen, T.: Haptic palpation for medical simulation in virtual environments. IEEE Trans. Vis. Comput. Graph. **18**(4), 617–625 (2012). https://doi.org/10.1109/tvcg.2012.46
629. Ullrich, S., Rausch, D., Kuhlen, T.W.: Bimanual haptic simulator for medical training: System architecture and performance measurements. In: Proceeding of Joint Virtual Reality Conference of EGVE—EuroVR, pp. 39–46 (2011). https://doi.org/10.2312/EGVE/JVRC11/039-046
630. van Unen, V., Höllt, T., Pezzotti, N., Li, N., Reinders, M.J.T., Eisemann, E., Koning, F., Vilanova, A., Lelieveldt, B.P.F.: Visual analysis of mass cytometry data by hierarchical stochastic neighbour embedding reveals rare cell types. Nat. Commun. **8**(1), 1740 (2017). https://doi.org/10.1038/s41467-017-01689-9

631. Vad, V., Byška, J., Jurčík, A., Viola, I., Gröller, E.M., Hauser, H., Marques, S.M., Damborský, J., Kozlíková, B.: Watergate: Visual exploration of water trajectories in protein dynamics. In: Proceeding of Eurographics Workshop on Visual Computing for Biology and Medicine, pp. 33–42 (2017). https://doi.org/10.2312/VCBM.20171235
632. Valentino, D., Mazziotta, J., Huang, H.: Visualization of human brain structure-function relationships. In: Proceeding of IEEE Engineering in Medicine and Biology, pp. 1737–1738 (1989). https://doi.org/10.1109/iembs.1989.96431
633. Valentino, D.J., Mazziotta, J.C., Huang, H.: Volume rendering of multimodal images: application to MRI and PET imaging of the human brain. IEEE Trans. Med. Imaging **10**(4), 554–562 (1991). https://doi.org/10.1109/42.108590
634. Van Der Zwan, M., Lueks, W., Bekker, H., Isenberg, T.: Illustrative molecular visualization with continuous abstraction. Comput. Graph. Forum **30**(3), 683–690 (2011). https://doi.org/10.1111/J.1467-8659.2011.01917.X
635. Van Pelt, R., Bescós, J.O., Breeuwer, M., Clough, R.E., Gröller, M.E., ter Haar Romenij, B., Vilanova, A.: Exploration of 4D MRI blood flow using stylistic visualization. IEEE Trans. Vis. Comput. Graph. **16**(6), 1339–1347 (2010). https://doi.org/10.1109/tvcg.2010.153
636. Van Pelt, R., Bescós, J.O., Breeuwer, M., Clough, R.E., Gröller, M.E., ter Haar Romenij, B., Vilanova, A.: Interactive virtual probing of 4D MRI blood-flow. IEEE Trans. Vis. Comput. Graph. **17**(12), 2153–2162 (2011). https://doi.org/10.1109/tvcg.2011.215
637. Varshney, A., Brooks, F., Richardson, D.C., Wright, W.V., Manocha, D.: Defining, computing, and visualizing molecular interfaces. In: Proceeding of IEEE Visualization, pp. 36–43 (1995). https://doi.org/10.1109/visual.1995.480793
638. Varshney, A., Brooks, F.P., Wright, W.V.: Computing smooth molecular surfaces. IEEE Comput. Graph. Appl. **14**(05), 19–25 (1994). https://doi.org/10.1109/38.310720
639. Vázquez, P.P., Götzelmann, T., Hartmann, K., Nürnberger, A.: An interactive 3D framework for anatomical education. Int. J. Comput. Assist. Radiol. Surg. **3**(6), 511–524 (2008). https://doi.org/10.1007/s11548-008-0251-4
640. Vázquez, P.P., Hermosilla, P., Guallar, V., Estrada, J., Vinacua, À.: Visual analysis of protein-ligand interactions. Comput. Graph. Forum **37**(3), 391–402 (2018). https://doi.org/10.1111/CGF.13428
641. Venter, J.C., Adams, M.D., Myers, E.W., Li, P.W., Mural, R.J., Sutton, G.G., Smith, H.O., Yandell, M., Evans, C.A., Holt, R.A., et al.: The sequence of the human genome. Science **291**(5507), 1304–1351 (2001). https://doi.org/10.1126/science.1058040
642. Vetter, C., Lasser, T., Okur, A., Navab, N.: 1D–3D registration for intra-operative nuclear imaging in radio-guided surgery. IEEE Trans. Med. Imaging **34**(2), 608–617 (2014). https://doi.org/10.1109/TMI.2014.2363551
643. Vilanova, A., Berenschot, G., Van Pul, C.: DTI visualization with streamsurfaces and evenly-spaced volume seeding. In: Proceeding of Eurographics/IEEE VGTC Symposium on Visualization, pp. 173–182 (2004). https://doi.org/10.2312/VISSYM/VISSYM04/173-182
644. Vilanova, A., Gröller, E.: Geometric modelling for virtual colon unfolding. In: Geometric Modeling for Scientific Visualization, pp. 453–468. Berlin, Heidelberg (2004). https://doi.org/10.1007/978-3-662-07443-527
645. Vilanova Bartroli, A., Wegenkittl, R., König, A., Gröller, E.: Nonlinear virtual colon unfolding. In: Proceeding of IEEE Visualization, pp. 411–418 (2001). https://doi.org/10.1109/visual.2001.964540
646. Viola, I., Gröller, M.E.: Smart visibility in visualization. In: Proceeding of Computational Aesthetics, pp. 209–216 (2005). https://doi.org/10.2312/COMPAESTH/COMPAESTH05/209-216

647. Vourvopoulos, A., Faria, A.L., Ponnam, K., Bermudez i Badia, S.: RehabCity: design and validation of a cognitive assessment and rehabilitation tool through gamified simulations of activities of daily living. In: Proceeding of Advances in Computer Entertainment Technology, pp. 1–8 (2014). https://doi.org/10.1145/2663806.2663852
648. Vrahatis, A.G., Tasoulis, S.K., Dimitrakopoulos, G.N., Plagianakos, V.P.: Visualizing high-dimensional single-cell RNA-seq data via random projections and geodesic distances. In: Proceeding of IEEE Conference on Computational Intelligence in Bioinformatics and Computational Biology (2019). https://doi.org/10.1109/cibcb.2019.8791482
649. Šoltészová, V., Patel, D., Bruckner, S., Viola, I.: A multidirectional occlusion shading model for direct volume rendering. Comput. Graph. Forum **29**(3), 883–891 (2010). https://doi.org/10.1111/j.1467-8659.2009.01695.x
650. Wagner, M., Slijepcevic, D., Horsak, B., Rind, A., Zeppelzauer, M., Aigner, W.: KAVAGait: knowledge-assisted visual analytics for clinical gait analysis. IEEE Trans. Vis. Comput. Graph. **25**(3), 1528–1542 (2018). https://doi.org/10.1109/TVCG.2017.2785271
651. Wagner, S., Illner, K., Weber, M., Preim, B., Saalfeld, P.: VR acrophobia treatment - development of customizable acrophobia inducing scenarios. In: Proceeding of Eurographics Workshop on Visual Computing for Biology and Medicine, pp. 49–53 (2020). https://doi.org/10.2312/VCBM.20201171
652. Wagner, S., Joeres, F., Gabele, M., Hansen, C., Preim, B., Saalfeld, P.: Difficulty factors for VR cognitive rehabilitation training-crossing a virtual road. Comput. Graph. **83**, 11–22 (2019). https://doi.org/10.1016/j.cag.2019.06.009
653. Wan, M., Liang, Z., Ke, Q., Hong, L., Bitter, I., Kaufman, A.: Automatic centerline extraction for virtual colonoscopy. IEEE Trans. Med. Imaging **21**(12), 1450–1460 (2002). https://doi.org/10.1109/tmi.2002.806409
654. Wan, M., Tang, Q., Kaufman, A., Liang, Z., Wax, M.: Volume rendering based interactive navigation within the human colon. In: Proceeding of IEEE Visualization, pp. 397–549 (1999). https://doi.org/10.1109/visual.1999.809914
655. Wang, C., Cheikh, F.A., Kaaniche, M., Elle, O.J.: Liver surface reconstruction for image guided surgery. In: Proceeding of SPIE Medical Imaging: Image-guided Procedures, Robotic Interventions, and Modeling, pp. 576–583 (2018). https://doi.org/10.1117/12.2297398
656. Wang, H., Chen, F., Zhang, L., Zhang, B., Pan, M., Wu, X., Tang, J.: Research on visualization of three-dimensional surface in tumor magnetic inductive thermotherapy plan system. In: Proceeding of IEEE Conference on Signal and Image Processing, pp. 925–929 (2020). https://doi.org/10.1109/ICSIP49896.2020.9339336
657. Wang, Q., Laramee, R.S.: EHR STAR: the state-of-the-art in interactive EHR visualization. Comput. Graph. Forum **41**(1), 69–105 (2022). https://doi.org/10.1111/CGF.14424
658. Wang, T.D., Plaisant, C., Quinn, A.J., Stanchak, R., Murphy, S., Shneiderman, B.: Aligning temporal data by sentinel events: discovering patterns in electronic health records. In: Proceeding of the CHI Conference on Human Factors in Computing Systems, pp. 457–466 (2008). https://doi.org/10.1145/1357054.1357129
659. Ward, J.W., Phillips, R., Bøjen, A., Grau, C., Jois, D., Beavis, A.W.: A virtual environment for radiotherapy training and education-VERT. In: Proceeding of Eurographics—Dirk Bartz Prize, pp. 5–8 (2011). https://doi.org/10.2312/EG2011/MED/005-008
660. Warrick, P.A., Funnell, W.R.J.: A VRML-based anatomical visualization tool for medical education. IEEE Trans. Inf. Technol. Biomed. **2**(2), 55–61 (1998). https://doi.org/10.1109/4233.720523
661. Wei, M., Wang, J., Guo, X., Wu, H., Xie, H., Wang, F.L., Qin, J.: Learning-based 3D surface optimization from medical image reconstruction. Opt. Lasers Eng. **103**, 110–118 (2018). https://doi.org/10.1016/j.optlaseng.2017.11.014

662. Wei, M., Zhu, L., Yu, J., Wang, J., Pang, W.M., Wu, J., Qin, J., Heng, P.A.: Morphology-preserving smoothing on polygonized isosurfaces of inhomogeneous binary volumes. Comput. Aided Des. **58**, 92–98 (2015). https://doi.org/10.1016/j.cad.2014.08.015
663. Weinstein, D., Kindlmann, G., Lundberg, E.: Tensorlines: Advection-diffusion based propagation through diffusion tensor fields. In: Proceeding of IEEE Visualization, pp. 249–530 (1999). https://doi.org/10.1109/visual.1999.809894
664. Weiss, P.L.T., Raban, D.R., Geifman, D., Keshner, E.A.: Dissemination of research in virtual reality-based rehabilitation: journal publication profiles. In: Proceeding of International Conference on Virtual Rehabilitation, pp. 1–6 (2019). https://doi.org/10.1109/icvr46560.2019.8994545
665. Wenger, A., Keefe, D.F., Zhang, S., Laidlaw, D.H.: Interactive volume rendering of thin thread structures within multivalued scientific data sets. IEEE Trans. Vis. Comput. Graph. **10**(6), 664–672 (2004). https://doi.org/10.1109/tvcg.2004.46
666. Wentzel, A., Hanula, P., Luciani, T., Elgohari, B., Elhalawani, H., Canahuate, G., Vock, D., Fuller, C.D., Marai, G.E.: Cohort-based T-SSIM visual computing for radiation therapy prediction and exploration. IEEE Trans. Vis. Comput. Graph. **26**(1), 949–959 (2019). https://doi.org/10.1109/tvcg.2019.2934546
667. Wesarg, S., Kirschner, M.: 3D visualization of medical image data employing 2D histograms. In: Proceeding of International Conference in Visualisation, pp. 153–158 (2009). https://doi.org/10.1109/VIZ.2009.30
668. Westenberg, M.A., van Hijum, S.A.F.T., Kuipers, O.P., Roerdink, J.B.T.M.: Visualizing genome expression and regulatory network dynamics in genomic and metabolic context. Comput. Graph. Forum **27**(3), 887–894 (2008). https://doi.org/10.1111/j.1467-8659.2008.01221.x
669. Westermann, B., Hauser, R.: Non-invasive 3-D patient registration for image-guided skull base surgery. Comput. Graph. **20**(6), 793–799 (1996). https://doi.org/10.1016/s0097-8493(96)00049-0
670. Wolf, F.A., Hamey, F.K., Plass, M., Solana, J., Dahlin, J.S., Göttgens, B., Rajewsky, N., Simon, L., Theis, F.J.: PAGA: graph abstraction reconciles clustering with trajectory inference through a topology preserving map of single cells. Genome Biol. **20**(1) (2019). https://doi.org/10.1186/s13059-019-1663-x
671. Wong, P.C., Wong, K.K., Foote, H., Thomas, J.: Global visualization and alignments of whole bacterial genomes. IEEE Trans. Vis. Comput. Graph. **9**(3), 361–377 (2003). https://doi.org/10.1109/TVCG.2003.1207444
672. Wongsuphasawat, K., Guerra Gómez, J.A., Plaisant, C., Wang, T.D., Taieb-Maimon, M., Shneiderman, B.: LifeFlow: visualizing an overview of event sequences. In: Proceeding of the CHI Conference on Human Factors in Computing Systems, pp. 1747–1756 (2011). https://doi.org/10.1145/1978942.1979196
673. Wooning, J., Benmahdjoub, M., van Walsum, T., Marroquim, R.: AR-assisted craniotomy planning for tumour resection. In: Proceeding of Eurographics Workshop on Visual Computing in Biology and Medicine, pp. 135–144 (2021). https://doi.org/10.2312/VCBM.20211353
674. Wrzesien, M., Alcañiz, M., Botella, C., Burkhardt, J.M., Bretón-López, J., Ortega, M., Brotons, D.B.: The therapeutic lamp: treating small-animal phobias. IEEE Comput. Graph. Appl. **33**(1), 80–86 (2013). https://doi.org/10.1109/MCG.2013.12
675. Wu, D., Roberge, J., Cork, D., Nguyen, B., Grace, T.: Computer visualization of long genomic sequences. In: Proceeding of IEEE Visualization, pp. 308–315 (1993). https://doi.org/10.1109/VISUAL.1993.398883
676. Wu, H.Y., Nöllenburg, M., Sousa, F.L., Viola, I.: Metabopolis: scalable network layout for biological pathway diagrams in urban map style. BMC Bioinf. **20**(1), 187 (2019). https://doi.org/10.1186/s12859-019-2779-4

677. Wu, H.Y., Nöllenburg, M., Viola, I.: Multi-level area balancing of clustered graphs. IEEE Trans. Vis. Comput. Graph. **28**(7), 2682–2696 (2020). https://doi.org/10.1109/TVCG.2020.3038154
678. Wu, J., Wei, M., Li, Y., Ma, X., Jia, F., Hu, Q.: Scale-adaptive surface modeling of vascular structures. Biomed. Eng. Online **9**(1), 75 (2010). https://doi.org/10.1186/1475-925X-9-75
679. Wu, Y., Tamayo, P., Zhang, K.: Visualizing and interpreting single-cell gene expression datasets with similarity weighted nonnegative embedding. Cell Syst. **7**(6), 656-666.e4 (2018). https://doi.org/10.1016/j.cels.2018.10.015
680. Yoo, T.S., Bliss, D., Lowekamp, B.C., Chen, D.T., Murphy, G.E., Narayan, K., Hartnell, L.M., Do, T., Subramaniam, S.: Visualizing cells and humans in 3D: biomedical image analysis at nanometer and meter scales. IEEE Comput. Graph. Appl. **32**(5), 39–49 (2012). https://doi.org/10.1109/MCG.2012.68
681. You, S., Hong, L., Wan, M., Junyaprasert, K., Kaufman, A., Muraki, S., Zhou, Y., Wax, M., Liang, Z.: Interactive volume rendering for virtual colonoscopy. In: Proceeding of IEEE Visualization, pp. 433–436 (1997). https://doi.org/10.1109/VISUAL.1997.663915
682. Zeng, W., Marino, J., Kaufman, A., Gu, X.D.: Volumetric colon wall unfolding using harmonic differentials. Comput. Graph. **35**(3), 726–732 (2011). https://doi.org/10.1016/j.cag.2011.03.008
683. Zhang, C., Höllt, T., Caan, M.W., Eisemann, E., Vilanova, A.: Comparative visualization for diffusion tensor imaging group study at multiple levels of detail. In: Proceeding of Eurographics Workshop on Visual Computing for Biology and Medicine, pp. 53–62 (2017). https://doi.org/10.2312/VCBM.20171237
684. Zhang, C., Schultz, T., Lawonn, K., Eisemann, E., Vilanova, A.: Glyph-based comparative visualization for diffusion tensor fields. IEEE Trans. Vis. Comput. Graph. **22**(1), 797–806 (2015). https://doi.org/10.1109/TVCG.2015.2467435
685. Zhang, G., Liu, X., Fox, M.D.: Visualization of ventricles of the brain by volume rendering. In: Proceeding of IEEE Engineering in Medicine and Biology, pp. 542–543 (1989). https://doi.org/10.1109/IEMBS.1989.95864
686. Zhang, Q., Karunanithi, M., Kang, C.: Immersive augmented reality (I am real)–remote clinical consultation. In: Proceeding of IEEE EMBS Conference on Biomedical and Health Informatics, pp. 1–4 (2019). https://doi.org/10.1109/bhi.2019.8834641
687. Zhang, S., Demiralp, C., Laidlaw, D.H.: Visualizing diffusion tensor MR images using streamtubes and streamsurfaces. IEEE Trans. Vis. Comput. Graph. **9**(4), 454–462 (2003). https://doi.org/10.1109/tvcg.2003.1260740
688. Zhao, L., van Ravesteijn, V.F., Botha, C.P., Truyen, R., Vos, F.M., Post, F.H.: Surface curvature line clustering for polyp detection in CT colonography. In: Proceeding of Eurographics Workshop on Visual Computing in Biology and Medicine, pp. 53–60 (2008). https://doi.org/10.2312/VCBM/VCBM08/053-060
689. Zheng, G.X.Y., Terry, J.M., Belgrader, P., Ryvkin, P., Bent, Z.W., Wilson, R., Ziraldo, S.B., Wheeler, T.D., et al.: Massively parallel digital transcriptional profiling of single cells. Nat. Commun. **8**(1) (2017). https://doi.org/10.1038/ncomms14049
690. Zuiderveld, K.J., Koning, A.H., Stokking, R., Maintz, J., Appelman, F.J., Viergever, M.A.: Multimodality visualization of medical volume data. Comput. Graph. **20**(6), 775–791 (1996). https://doi.org/10.1016/S0097-8493(96)00050-7

MIX
Papier aus verantwortungsvollen Quellen
Paper from responsible sources
FSC® C105338

If you have any concerns about our products,
you can contact us on
ProductSafety@springernature.com

In case Publisher is established outside the EU,
the EU authorized representative is:
Springer Nature Customer Service Center GmbH
Europaplatz 3, 69115 Heidelberg, Germany

Printed by Libri Plureos GmbH
in Hamburg, Germany